MEA

MW01232787

This book includes:

Bodybuilding, Weight Loss. Beginners Guide to Detox your Body with Intermittent Fasting. Quick and Easy Recipes to Burn Fast, Lose Weight Incorporating Anti Aging Nutrients into the Diet.

Michell Peterson

Table of Contents

Meal Prep for Bodybuilding

Meal Prep for Weight Loss

Meal Prep For Bodybuilding

A Healthy Nutrition Prep Guide to Follow Right Diet, Grow Muscle and Stay Motivated. Learn How to Make "Ready to Go" Meals to Burn Extra Fats.

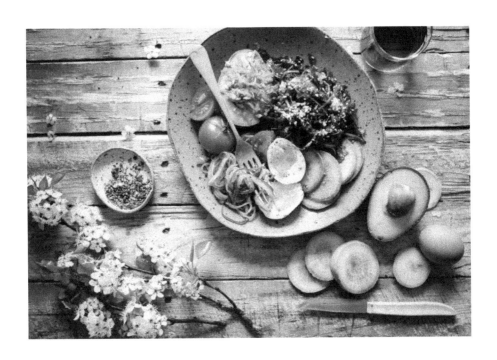

Introduction

It's simple stuff really, but with bodybuilding and dieting in general, we all tend to overcomplicate things. Once you have your diet plan in place, it becomes so much easier to build your shopping list each week.

Bodybuilding is a science, and if you understand how it works, you will be able to get ripped in no time – that is, if you put in the work, of course. This book is not about the workouts though. It is about the diet that you need to complement your bodybuilding activities and get those gains. Success in bodybuilding does not come through training alone.

There are various factors to consider in bodybuilding: the right measurement, the proper training, the duration of training, the diet, supplements to take, ensuring recovery after workout, and staying motivated, among others. Given all these considerations, it is obvious that bodybuilding requires focus and discipline not only in the way the bodybuilder trains but also in terms of what he eats and drinks.

It is important to realize what value nutrition holds for the muscles. Before you even think about the kind of weight training to do, you have to understand how your muscles develop and what nutrients they need. There are different views on nutrition and bodybuilding, varying depending on the expertise and specialization of the person giving out advice. Three common factors are identified as essential in building muscles: training, supplementation, and diet. When all these are properly done, the body builder can expect to see optimum results within a short period of time.

The goals of bodybuilding can never be truly achieved through weightlifting exercises alone. Diet plays a significant role in realizing your bodybuilding goals. In bodybuilding, it is necessary that you accompany exercises with proper diet and nutrition. I will inform you about the nutrients that your body needs for bodybuilding. At the same time, you will find examples of the kinds of food that contain these nutrients to serve as a guide in making your nutrition plan.

You've probably heard of meal prepping before but you may be confused on what it really means. Do you prep the meal the hour before, the day before, the week before? How is it done? These are some common and very relevant questions.

Meal prepping is when you make all your meals in advance for the next week or a certain amount of time. Meal prepping can be done by either cooking all your food one day for the rest of the week, or it can be done by assembling all your meals to freeze them for the next month! Either way is a great way to meal prep, they just require different steps. The best part of meal prepping is that it isn't a one-size fit all package. You get to choose how often you meal prep and for how many meals you want to meal prep. Maybe one week you want to meal prep all of your meals and the next week just breakfast. This is doable! Your meal prep journey is completely up to you.

Chapter 1   Meal Prepping

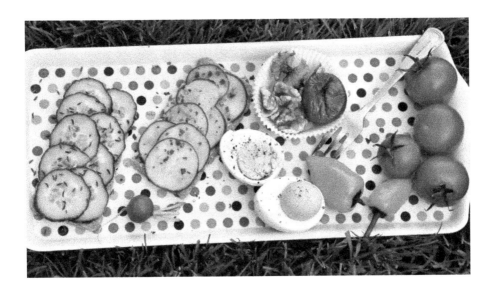

We are busy. There is no way around it, but we still need to provide our families with healthy homemade meals. That is why so many people are turning to meal prepping. Meal prepping is going to allow you to eliminate some of the stress from your life by ensuring that you do not have to cook a meal from scratch every single night. Meal prepping also helps you to reduce the amount of time that you are in the kitchen and it can help keep you healthy as well.

You can choose to just meal prep your dinners, or you can do breakfast, lunch, and dinner as well as snacks If you want. The number of meals that you choose to prep is completely up to you and it will all depend on how much time you want to dedicate each week to prepping. Meal prepping is basically preparing the food that you are going to eat ahead of time so that you can stick to a specific diet or schedule. Cooked foods, as well as raw foods, are included in meal prepping. There are many different ways to use meal prepping and many different benefits as well.

One of the things that hits people the hardest when they are trying to eat healthily or include more home cooked meals is the amount of time that they have to spend cooking, however, meal prepping can reduce this drastically because most of the cooking is done on one day of the week.

Meal prepping is a great way to help you find a bit of balance in your life by taking just a bit of time at the start of the week, you will find that you have a lot more time during the rest of the week to do the things you enjoy.

Why Meal Prep?

People choose to meal prep for many different reasons. Some choose to meal prep because they want to live a healthy lifestyle. They want to have the energy that comes with eating healthy, but because life is so busy they find it hard to take the time each day to make their meals. Meal prepping ensures that they are able to stay consistent which helps them to reach their goals. Another reason that people choose to meal prep is because they are busy and the idea of coming home after a long day at work just to stand over the stove and cook a meal is overwhelming. It is usually time that determines what they are eating, which leads us to the third reason.

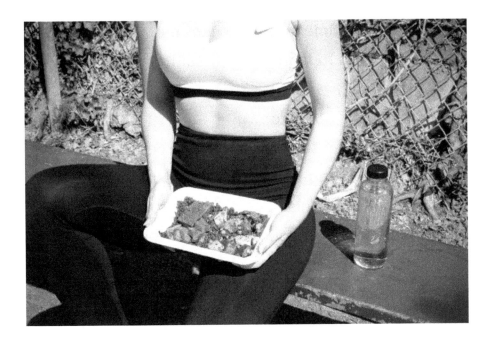

The third reason that many people choose to meal prep is because they are tired of picking food up through the drive thru, ordering out, spending far too much money on food, and putting unhealthy foods into their bodies. Meal prep simply means meal preparation, which is simply planning your meals, preparing them and packaging them for the upcoming days. Most people that meal prep will prepare meals a week in advance, however, those that use the freezer meal system can prep their meals up to a month in advance.

You will prep your meals according to what works best for you and your family. The goal of meal prepping is not just to save time in the kitchen, but also to ensure you have access to homemade, healthy meals every day of the week.

Meal prepping is going to:

- Help you save money. Many people believe that eating healthy is more expensive, however, this does not have to be the case, especially if you meal prep. When you meal prep, you are going to buy some of your foods in bulk. This is going to save you a ton of money. On top of that, you are going to know exactly what meals you are going to create which is going to give you a plan when you go to the grocery store. When you walk in with a plan, you are going to know exactly what you need to purchase instead of wandering aimlessly or returning to the store several times during the week to grab extra ingredients. As if that was not enough, when you meal prep your lunches, you are going to cut your cost because you will not be going out to pick up expensive food when you are on your lunch break.

- Meal prepping is going to help you lose weight. Knowing what you are going to eat is very important if you want to lose weight. Meal prepping is going to help ensure that you know exactly what is going into your body and it is going to help with portion control. You are going to know in advance how many calories you are eating and you are going to feel more energetic because you are eating healthy foods.
- When you meal prep, you are going to find that grocery shopping is much easier for you. Each week, you are going to be able to walk into the grocery store with your list and know exactly what you need to purchase. This is

going to reduce impulse buys and help you avoid areas of the store such as the cookie aisle where you are tempted.

- Meal prepping is going to help you control the portions of the meals that you are eating. When your meals are already packaged and ready to go, it reduces the chances that you are going to go back and get more.

- Reducing waste is a huge benefit of meal prepping. How many times have you had to throw out food because it has gone bad in your fridge? When you meal prep, you are going to make sure that you use up all of your ingredients, each week and if you plan correctly, there are going to be no leftovers to go bad.

- Meal prepping is a huge time saver. You will have to spend some time once a week, creating your meal plan and grocery list as well as prepping your meals, but overall, you are going to save a ton of time. Think about how much time you have wasted trying to figure out what you should cook. Think about all of the time, that you spend each night standing in front of the stove or cleaning up after you cook a meal. All of that is done once and all you have to do is heat your food up.

- When you meal prep, you are investing in your own health. Because you are going to be choosing what you will eat in advance, it is very likely that you will eat healthier, cleaner meals than people who do not practice meal prepping. Of course, eating healthy will lead to weight loss, but more importantly, it will lead to a healthy body.

- Cravings are going to stop as you continue to meal prep. In just a few weeks, you will find that you no longer crave sugar or junk. Instead, you will be looking forward to the meals and snacks that you have prepared.

- Stress is a killer. It can cause so many problems with your health such as increasing your blood pressure. It can cause sleep issues, lower your immune system, and even cause digestive problems. Meal planning can reduce some of the stress in your life and allow you a bit of time to relax each day. It is great to know that when you come home after work, your food is already prepared and ready for you to eat.

- Meal prepping is going to ensure that you are eating a variety of foods and that your body is getting the nutrition that it needs. You don't have to eat the same meals every single week, mix it up and try out some new recipes.

Chapter 2   Essential Bodybuilding Nutrition
For Meal Preppers

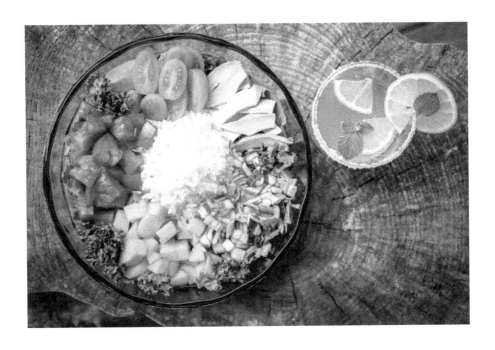

Education is helpful for those times when you may wonder how all your efforts are going to pay off. I know we've covered macros to an extent already, but now let's take a deeper look. The more educated you are about how the right balance of protein, carbs, and fats can get you the body you're working toward, the more likely you'll be to stick with the program. Knowledge is power, right?

Macros

The three macronutrients that make up all (yes, literally all) foods are protein, carbohydrates, and fat. Your body has different purposes for each.

PROTEIN

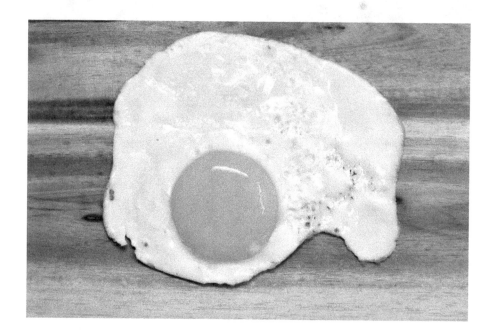

let's start with protein. After all, it's every bodybuilder's favorite macro, and for good reason. Protein from the food we eat really does live up to its reputation for building muscle.

As you put stress on your muscles through lifting, you actually create microscopic tears in the muscle fibers that need to be rebuilt. That's when the protein from your diet rushes in to repair those areas, ultimately building them back up to be larger and stronger. Protein also serves numerous other functions in the body, from giving cells their structure to serving as the backbone of hormones and enzymes.

Most sedentary people need an average of 1.2 to 1.8 grams of protein per kilogram of body weight (0.54 to 0.82 grams per pound) to stay healthy—but if you've picked up this book, I'm guessing you wouldn't classify yourself as sedentary. In my experience, and based on the latest research, someone who's lifting on a regular basis requires anywhere from 1.8 to 3.3 grams of protein per kilogram of body weight (0.8 to 1.5 grams per pound).

Some favorite sources of protein for bodybuilders include lean ground beef, chicken, salmon, whitefish, turkey, eggs, Greek yogurt, cottage cheese, tofu, beans, and protein powder.

PLANT-BASED PROTEIN

Throughout this book, I've provided several recipes built around plant-based protein. If you're more the meat-and-potatoes type, you may not have experimented much with protein from plants. I'd like to encourage you to keep an open mind, though, as nutrition science increasingly shows that a diet full of plants has numerous advantages for health, from reducing the risk of cancer and heart disease to helping maintain a healthy weight.

If you're concerned that going with less meat could keep you from bulking, you can set those worries aside. With proper meal planning, you can still reach your goals on a plant-based diet. You just have to make sure to consume enough protein.

Some additional bonuses of plant sources of protein include fiber, vitamins, and minerals. Plant-based protein also typically contains less saturated fat than animal-based protein. Excellent choices for plant-based protein include beans, lentils, nuts and nut butters, quinoa and other grains, and soy foods like tofu, tempeh, and edamame.

And meat lovers, never fear. I've included plenty of straight-up meat dishes throughout this book as well. You can expect to find recipes for beef, pork, chicken, and turkey throughout.

CARBS

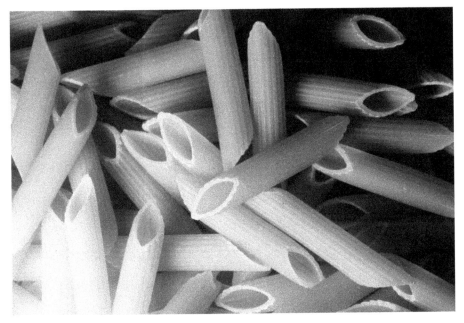

While it's popular these days to stay away from carbohydrates to keep a svelte figure, there's definitely a point where low-carb can be overdone—or even dangerous. Here's the thing: Your brain runs on glucose, the broken-down form of carbohydrates. So without enough of these critical macros, you can begin to feel mentally foggy. What's more, carbohydrates are the body's preferred energy source, meaning that skimping on them can lead to serious fatigue—the last thing you want when you're headed to the gym for a challenging lifting workout.

Foods that contain carbohydrates also typically provide fiber, a much-needed nutrient for digestion and disease prevention. Carbohydrates also boast numerous vitamins, minerals, and antioxidants you just won't find in a protein-packed steak all by itself.

The key for choosing the best carbohydrates to meet your bodybuilding goals is to mainly stick with complex, minimally processed carbs. Examples include beans; whole grains like quinoa, oats, barley, brown rice, and whole-wheat bread; veggies like squash, potatoes, carrots, and corn; and fruits like apples, berries, and bananas.

FAT

There was a time (remember the nineties?) when we believed that dietary fat made us fat. But research has come a long way and shown that this simply isn't the case. In fact, fat serves many critical purposes in the body (and thank goodness, because otherwise we'd still be eating those terrible fat-free cookies!).

Fat in our foods gets converted in the body to keep us warm, provide protective cushioning for our organs, help us absorb certain nutrients, and—my favorite—help us stay fuller longer. When you're working on bulking, adding extra fat is an easy way to consume more calories, since fat contains five more calories per gram than protein and carbohydrates.

Still, just like the other macros, not all fats are created equal. While science is still working to pin down exactly the right amount of saturated fat and cholesterol that are good for health, we know that certain fat sources have evidence-based benefits.

Some of the best choices for fat sources include fatty fish like salmon and sardines, eggs, nuts and nut butters, olives, avocados, full-fat yogurt and cheese, chia seeds and flaxseed, and olive, coconut, and avocado oils.

Make Your Meals Work for You

When you're working toward bodybuilding goals, food is your fuel. And just like you fill your car's tank with high-quality gas to make it run smoothly, you want to fill your body with the best sources of energy and nutrients possible. Here's how each meal of the day can help you see results.

BREAKFAST

Breakfast may or may not be the most important meal of the day, depending on who you ask, but it is an opportunity to start your day with excellent nutrition. If you're among those who like to time your workouts early in the morning, breakfast will play a critical role in supporting your training, whether as your pre-workout fuel or your post-workout recovery.

LUNCH

When you've got a busy, on-the-go lifestyle, it can be tempting to occasionally skip lunch—but resist the temptation. Your body needs to stay fueled throughout the day. Having a healthy lunch keeps you from bingeing on lower-quality foods (aka processed junk) later. Plus, if you're working out in the afternoon, your lunch can serve as your pre-workout meal and will help ensure that you bring the proper level of intensity and energy to the gym.

DINNER

For many of us, dinner is when we consume the most calories, so this meal is really "where the magic happens." As you progress through your meal prepping program, you'll find the recipes provided in this book will balance your macros for the best results. At dinner, you'll be eating high protein (to keep your body building muscle, especially as you get leaner), low to moderate fat (to keep you full, help absorb nutrients, and assist with proper hormone production), and varying levels of carbs (based on your bodybuilding goals and daily activity levels).

SNACKS

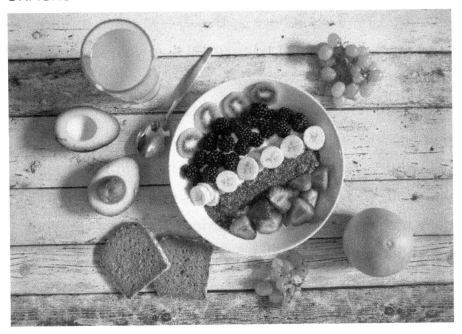

Who doesn't love to snack? I'm all for breaking up the day with small bursts of calories and macros. Doing so helps keep blood sugar steady, meaning you'll feel less hungry and have the energy you need around your workouts. And the right choice of snacks can help you reach your calorie targets if you're working on bulking.

CHEAT MEAL

You've probably heard a lot of varying opinions about the concept of a "cheat meal." My stance is to leave this decision up to you. The occasional extra indulgence certainly isn't going to be a deal-breaker for reaching your bodybuilding goals. So if you feel the need to have a comfort food meal here or there, or a piece of dark chocolate every day, I hope you'll give yourself the freedom to do so.

The good news about counting macros, or following an If It Fits in Your Macros (IIFYM) style of diet, as we are doing here, is that with just a little bit of foresight and planning, you can easily work these meals into your daily macronutrient targets without straying from your bodybuilding goals. A high-carb, high-fat mac and cheese or chocolate cake, for example, could be balanced out later with lower-fat, higher-protein choices combined with some low-calorie, low-carb veggies.

Goals & Dietary Needs

Not everyone gets into bodybuilding with the same goals, and often your goals will change as time goes by. Typically, bodybuilding follows one of three paths: cutting, bulking, or maintaining.

Cutting means shedding body fat to get lean and toned. This phase of bodybuilding usually means cutting back on calories to allow your muscles to attain the definition you can show off during competition (or swimsuit) season.

Bulking, on the other hand, means training heavier for bigger muscle gains, which is usually accompanied by an increase in calories to support all the hard work you're putting in at the gym. And maintaining is, of course, when you stay the course to keep whatever physique you've got.

I understand that you may not be in the same phase as the person at the weight bench next to you. That's why you'll find the recipes in this meal prep plan to be highly customizable. Every week of meal plans can be tailored to any goal you're currently working toward.

The beauty of IIFYM is that you can set up your diet based on your own food preferences and tolerances, cooking ability, goals, and schedule and enjoy your favorite foods in moderation without feeling guilty or deprived. You can work treats and nontraditional diet foods into your plan without feeling guilty or panicking and falling completely off the rails. This is what a sustainable lifestyle looks like.

Now, here's where the cool, nitty-gritty, figuring out your specific caloric and macronutrient needs comes in, along with a few maybe not-so-fun math calculations. I promise I'll make it as simple and painless as possible. For the first calculation, you will need to know your weight, your approximate body fat percentage, and your activity level. With these numbers in hand, you will be able to figure out your Total Daily Energy

Expenditure (TDEE), which is the total amount of calories you burn over the course of a day (24 hours). To calculate your TDEE, you first need to calculate your Basal Metabolic Rate (BMR). There are several formulas you can use to do this, but my personal favorite for bodybuilders, who tend to have more muscle mass, is the Katch-McArdle formula, because it accounts for differences in body composition.

BMR = 370 + (21.6 x Lean Body Mass in KG)

BMR = 370 + (9.8 x Lean Body Mass in LB)

The one catch, of course, is that you have to know what your Lean Body Mass (LBM) is. If you don't know your LBM, you can use simpler (albeit less accurate) equations out there, like the Harris-Benedict or Mifflin-St Jeor. You can find many calculators online that will calculate it for you, as well as a formula (different for men and women). Just remember, whatever formula you choose, know that it simply provides you with an estimate as a starting point and may very well need to be adjusted once you test it out in real life.

Once you have calculated your BMR, you will need to add your additional energy expenditure based on your daily activity level. I have found that the standard Katch-McArdle activity multiplier tends to overestimate the amount of calories burned, so I use the below modified version to calculate activity levels.

Sedentary   Little to no exercise   BMR X 1.15

Light

Activity   Light exercise or sports

1 to 3 days per week   BMR X 1.2

Moderate

Activity   Moderate exercise or sports

3 to 5 days per week   BMR X 1.4

Very

Active   Hard exercise or sports

6 to 7 days per week   BMR X 1.6

Extra

Active   Extra-hard exercise or sports

6 to 7 days per week   BMR X 1.8

Super

Active   Extra-hard exercise or sports

6 to 7 days per week and a physical job BMR X 1.9

Remember that your TDEE is only a starting point and will likely need to be adjusted up or down based on the intensity and type of activity you engage in. If you're cutting, eat 75 to 80 percent of your TDEE, which is equivalent to a 20 to 25 percent caloric deficit. If you're bulking, eat 105 to 110 percent of your TDEE, which is equivalent to a 5 to 10 percent caloric surplus. Please note that I don't recommend bulking unless you're a male already at 10 percent body fat or less or a female already at 20 percent body fat or less.

MAINTAINING

Here's how to calculate your calories and macros if you're maintaining:

•TDEE x 1 = Daily Calories for Maintaining

•Set your protein intake to 0.8 to 1 grams per pound of body weight.

»Protein in grams/day = Body weight in pounds x 0.8 to 1

»Protein in grams/day x 4 = Daily Calories Coming from Protein

•Set your fat intake to 0.3 to 0.4 grams per pound of body weight.

»Fat in grams/day = Body weight in pounds x 0.3 to 0.4

»Fat in grams/day x 9 = Daily Calories Coming from Fat

•Set your carb intake to whatever calories remain.

»Add together your Daily Calories Coming from Protein and your Daily Calories Coming from Fat.

»Subtract this number from your Daily Calories for Cutting to get your Daily Calories Coming from Carbs.

»Divide your Daily Calories Coming from Carbs by 4 to calculate your Carbs in grams/day.

CUTTING

Here's how to calculate your calories and macros if you're cutting:

•TDEE x 0.75 to 0.8 = Daily Calories for Cutting

•Set your protein intake to 1 to 1.2 grams per pound of body weight.

»Protein in grams/day = Body weight in pounds x 1 to 1.2

»Protein in grams/day x 4 = Daily Calories Coming from Protein

•Set your fat intake to 0.2 to 0.25 grams per pound of body weight.

»Fat in grams/day = Body weight in pounds x 0.2 to 0.25

»Fat in grams/day x 9 = Daily Calories Coming from Fat

•Set your carb intake to whatever calories remain.

»Add together your Daily Calories Coming from Protein and your Daily Calories Coming from Fat.

»Subtract this number from your Daily Calories for Cutting to get your Daily Calories Coming from Carbs.

»Divide your Daily Calories Coming from Carbs by 4 to calculate your Carbs in grams/day.

BULKING

Here's how to calculate your calories and macros if you're bulking:

•TDEE x 1.05 to 1.10 = Daily Calories for Bulking

•Set your protein intake to 1 gram per pound of body weight.

»Protein in grams/day = Body weight in pounds x 1 to 1.2

»Protein in grams x 4 = Daily Calories Coming from Protein

•Set your fat intake to 0.3 to 0.4 grams per pound of body weight.

»Fat in grams/day = Body weight in pounds x 0.3 to 0.4

»Fat in grams x 9 = Daily Calories Coming from Fat

•Set your carb intake to whatever calories remain.

»Add together your Daily Calories Coming from Protein and your Daily Calories Coming from Fat.

»Subtract this number from your Daily Calories for Cutting to get your Daily Calories Coming from Carbs.

»Divide your Daily Calories Coming from Carbs by 4 to calculate your daily carbs in grams.

Please note that the above caloric and macronutrient requirements are only estimates and may need to be adjusted based on your metabolic rate, health, and a variety of lifestyle factors. So listen to your body, and make adjustments as needed based on how your body responds.

Tracking Macros

Now that you've completed your individualized daily caloric and macronutrient requirements, you're ready to start tracking your macros. You will need to be diligent, weighing or measuring what you eat and recording it in a food-tracking or meal-planning app. There are some great ones out there that scan barcodes and input macros for you automatically.

Changing the way you eat and think about food can be a challenge. Be patient and kind with yourself, and try not to be disappointed with your starting results. Although there are no quick fixes or shortcuts, if you're consistent with meeting your macros, a flex diet will allow you to eat the foods you enjoy for the rest of your life and still get the results you've always dreamed of.

Chapter 3   Principles and rules

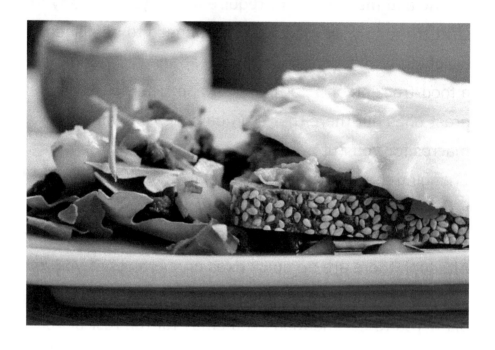

Here are the five must-know tips:

Pick your meals (3-5 days ahead of time)

Before shopping and prepping, you'll need to know what your meals that week will be. Depending on what your goals are, you can pick as many meals (breakfast, lunch, and dinner) as you want. If you have specific calorie goals in mind for each day, you will need to know all your snacks, too, if you want to be precise.

Think simple

This way, you don't have to stress about complicated cooking processes, getting a bunch of different ingredients at the store, or feeling overwhelmed about counting up calories and macronutrients. When you think simple, you can make a few different meals from staples like eggs, chicken, and vegetables.

Prep on a specific day

Rather than prep throughout the week, it's much more efficient to pick one day and prep most of your meals then. A lot of people choose Sunday, but whatever day you can free up works. If you're concerned about the amount of work and time prep takes, you can save some of the prep for the middle of the week on an evening when you have time.

Be ready to multitask

To speed up the prepping process, get ready to do some multi-tasking. You'll be cooking multiple things at once, and using your oven, stovetop, slow cooker, and any other equipment you have, like a pressure cooker. You can cook multiple things in the oven that have similar temperature and time requirements. Writing out the times, temperatures, and cooking method of what you're making can help you stay organized.

When meal prepping, you should pick your meals 3-5 days in advance, choose simple recipes, prep on a specific day, and learn to multitask.

Have the right containers

A common refrain of meal-prep articles and blogs is that the right containers are essential to productive meal-prepping. If your food isn't stored properly, it can go bad, dry out, get freezer-burn, and so on. Containers are so important that in the next section, we're going to take the time to break down what makes a container the right one.

Resources

Where are you going to find out how to meal prep and what recipes to make? While hopefully, this book is your number one resource, it's understandable if you still have a question here or there. We might not be able to guess all the questions you have (though we surely cracked our brains and try our best too!) or can't list everything there is to know about meal prepping in this book. Also, this book doesn't have all the meal prep recipes in the world! So, where do you go from here? Where can you get questions answered and find more recipes? One word, Google!

If you search online for meal prep questions or recipes, you'll be bombarded with hundreds of thousands of options and different websites. It can be overwhelming, which is why this book is so great to have. However, when you're looking for more recipes, there are plentiful online recipes that are delicious and nutritious! Always remember to look at the nutrition facts so that you aren't eating something that may look healthy but actually is not. Pinterest is a website that is a great source for meal prepping. If you aren't familiar with the social networking site, Pinterest now is the time to get acquainted. You can look at lots of different recipes according to your diet. There are gluten frees recipes, dairy-free recipes, and vegetarian, vegan, and paleo recipes too! If you are looking for specific recipes, definitely look no further than Pinterest. The most exciting feature about Pinterest is that you can save each recipe and organize them into different boards. Think of it as your new online cookbook! There are no limits to the amount of meal prep recipes you will be able to find.

If you would rather have more books in hand, there are tons of cookbooks that focus on meal prepping. This might be slightly more challenging, however, if you have dietary restrictions. We also have a large selection of recipes later on this book that you can pull from. You can make these recipes the start of your meal prep and add in more recipes once you feel you have mastered the ones here.

Food Storage

No one wants his or her food to spoil! Did you know that if your containers are not truly airtight then it could lead to your food going bad much more rapidly? A great recipe is only as good as what it is stored in! Food storage is one of the most important aspects of meal prep. Think of it as another addition to your cooking equipment. If you don't store your food properly, it will spoil quickly and leave your fridge with an unattractive odor that can stink your other food. This is especially important if you are cooking ahead your meals and portioning them out. You will need a lot more containers than normal so be ready to invest in some high-quality containers.

Save yourself more trouble and get a good quality set of food storage items. Food storage containers that are cheap typically comes with low-quality sealing materials that do not last very long and leave you spending more money in the long run as you have to replace them.

Plastic Food Sealing Bags

The first item for food storage you will need is plastic food sealing bags. Plastic food sealing bags are about to become your best friend! Plastic sealing bags of all different sizes are great to portion out your snacks or take some breakfast on the go. Ziploc food bags are good options. For your snack and breakfast, try to get sandwich-sized sealing bags. This will help you to be able to quickly grab your snacks as you head out the door. The best part about sandwich-sized bags is you can squeeze out the air and make them airtight to ensure your food stays fresh! You won't need these plastic bags for meals; these are only going to be used for snacks or breakfast items like muffins.

Plastic Freezer Bags

In addition to sandwich-sized plastic sealing bags, you'll also need gallon-sized freezer bags. When you prep your freezer meals, gallon size bags are an absolute must. They are super easy to write on with a permanent marker so that you won't forget how to cook it and how long to cook it. You can also write the name of the recipe on the gallon size bag so you can easily find the recipe you are searching for. Don't forget to write down the date you froze the recipe so you know to consume it within a 4-month period before turning bad. As a great tip to share on storing your freezer meals, you can squeeze out the air and lay them flat in your freezer so that they occupy minimal space. Then you can stack freezer meals on top of each other in order of "First in First Out" rule to keep your fridge organized and have your frozen food ingredients easily accessible.

Plastic and Glass Food Containers

For the days that you cook everything for the week in advance, solid storage containers are not to be missed. The last thing you need is for all your prepped meals to go bad because your containers were not up to requirements. There are two different types of containers to get. You can have glass or plastic storage containers. Stay away from stainless steel containers. While they make great storage containers, you cannot microwave them and so they don't have much of a place in a meal prep household.

Make sure to get a few different sized containers so that you portion each meal correctly and don't run out of the room. Whether you choose to use glass containers or plastic containers, it's a personal preference. While plastic may cheaper than glass, some people are afraid that the chemicals in the plastic can leach into your food while you reheat it. Plastic containers can also warp easily in the dishwasher. If your containers have warped, they need to be thrown out because they are no longer airtight. Glass doesn't stain, is easy to clean, and doesn't keep odors like plastic might. But while glass containers ensure that the chemicals from plastic don't leach into your food, they can be a little heavy to carry around. Glass will last longer than plastic if you do not drop them. Weigh the pros and cons of the two different types of containers and choose the option that best works for your lifestyle.

Food Vacuum Sealer Bags

If you want to buy in bulk and keep your meats as fresh as possible, vacuum-sealed bags can help with this. Vacuum sealer bags take out all the air from the bag so your food stays fresh longer. Keeping food fresh isn't their only benefit. When you vacuum seals your food, it saves you space. It makes the bag go so tightly around your prepped meal or meat that you do not need to worry about freezer space. This is a great addition if you are doing the freezer style meal prep. You can use vacuum bags of the similar required size for your portioning and this helps so much in organizing your freezer as well.

There are plenty of brands for Food Vacuum Sealing system selling in the market. Food Saver is one of the more popular and reliable brands that you may consider. It offers very decent sealing result and the food stored can last 2 to 3 times longer as compared to non-vacuum sealing methods in the freezer.

Cooking Wares

If you are cooking frequently, chances are you have an arsenal of cooking equipment that you already use at your disposal. However, if you are just starting out your cooking affairs, you may have little to nothing for your kitchen. This is especially true for new college students or newly-wed couples. With meal prepping, you will need a few different types of equipment to cook with. The good news is meal prepping doesn't require anything special in the kitchen. Everything you will buy can be used over and over or all you're cooking needs! It's time to go shopping!

Measuring Cups and Spoons

The most basic item required is a set of measuring cups and measuring spoons. You are going to be cooking a lot of different recipes and a good recipe depends on measurements. If you try to guess the measurements in a recipe, you'll end up with a less than desired meal. These measuring cups do not need to be anything fancy, grab the cheapest pair you can find and those will work! Make sure to have a set of cups that go from 1/4 cup to 1 cup, and a set of spoons that go from ¼ teaspoon to 1 tablespoon. You can find measuring cups and spoons at any grocery store and even at the dollar store.

Besides the measuring cups and spoons, you'll also need a few cooking utensils. Your cooking utensils will make your cooking go much easier and enjoyable. You don't want to be caught without a few good spatulas. Look for a spatula that you can use to scrape the sides of bowls for sauces and mixes. You'll also need a spatula that you can turn and lift with (the kind you need for pancakes!). In addition to these two spatulas, make sure you have other basic utensils like a whisk, a ladle, and a serving spoon.

Cooking Pots and Pans

You can't cook without items for the stove and oven! Let's talk about pots and pans. A good set of pots and pans is surely a great asset for an aspiring meal prepper. You'll be cooking a lot! Our favorite pan is a trusty cast-iron skillet. Cast iron skillets are cheap but they last forever. They hold their heat amazingly well and are great non-stick pans once they are seasoned correctly. They also create the perfect sear and greatly mimic a grill if you want grilled chicken or a hearty steak. They can also be placed in the oven to help you roast veggies and meats as well. And the best part about them is that they aren't too expensive! You can get a great cast iron skillet for around $25. Make sure you have at least two skillets and two pots. The pots will be used for cooking your grains and for steaming your veggies. They can also be used to make your sauces. You can use any pots you already may have but we recommend having a smaller saucepan and a pot large enough to cook your grains.

Knives and Cutting Equipment

If you plan on eating healthy, there's one kitchen tool you absolutely must have: a knife set. Meal prepping really cannot be done without a good knife set. You are going to be chopping up a ton of fruits and vegetables so make sure you have a trusty knife set and a few different cutting boards. There are a lot of different types of knives and multiple materials knives are made from. Stainless steel knives are sharp, easy to use, and heavy-duty. If you have a set of stainless-steel knives, there's no reason to replace them! If you haven't purchased a knife set yet, be aware that stainless steel can rust. Ceramic knives are a lot lighter than your traditional steel and they are super sharp. Just make sure you know what you are doing before you start chopping with ceramic. Ceramic knives can shatter if dropped or cut through something too hard. They are fairly cheap and they do not rust so they make a great choice if you want to try something new. If you don't want to buy a whole knife set, make sure you have at least the basic knives. Make sure to have a chef knife, a knife with a serrated edge, and a boning knife. We also recommend that you have a vegetable peeler. You may need to peel vegetables like potatoes, sweet potatoes, and squashes so we recommend you do not skip purchasing a vegetable peeler. You don't have to spend hundreds of dollars on new knives; you can get a new set of knives for around $50 that will certainly last you a while.

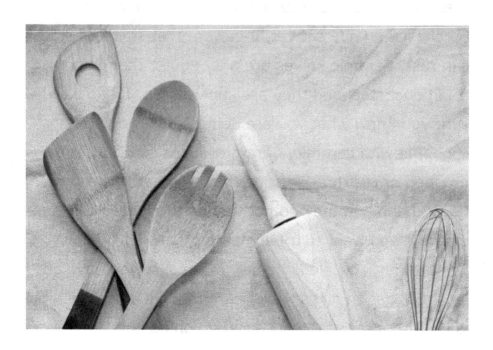

Oven Wares

You didn't think you could meal prep without roasting items, did you? Here comes that trusty cookie sheet! A cookie sheet is an absolute must with meal prepping. We use cookie sheets to roast our veggies then cook our protein on days we aren't using our pots/pans/slow cookers. An average size cookie sheet (size 13"x18") will be large enough to successfully cook whatever you need to. You can get a silicone baking mat to accompany your cookie sheet or just use parchment paper. This will help you save time on clean up and you won't have to scrub the cookie sheet after every single use. The baking mat and parchment paper are optional, but you will appreciate it after trying cooking without it.

Cooking Equipment

With all the wonderful recipes researched and ingredients nicely prepared, you're going to have it cooked. Different recipes call for different cooking methods thus the cooking apparatus varies. The following section brings to you the various cooking apparatus and explains how they can be used efficiently in your meal prep journey.

Stove Top & Induction Cooktop

To sauté, boil, fry, or steam, you will need a stovetop. Your stove can either be gas, electric, or induction. Most homes will come equipped with a few different sized stovetops. However, if you do not have a home that comes with a stovetop, you can buy a portable induction cooktop. These can be as small as a single stovetop and you can purchase one for around $50. You won't be able to meal prep without it.

Slow Cooker

If you are planning on doing any freezer meal prep, your most important tool is going to be your slow cooker. If you don't have a slow cooker, go out and buy one, it's about to become your new best friend! Slow cookers are extremely versatile and you can buy a new one for as little as $15. Slow cookers will make your meals taste like a million dollars without you lifting a finger. Even if you aren't planning on doing any freezer meals, a slow cooker can help you out with your prep work. You can put protein in the slow cooker in the morning and a few hours later you have tender and amazing meat for the rest of the week. This is one piece of equipment you won't regret buying.

Convection Oven

Convection ovens are great little tools. They can be set up on your counter but will be able to bake or roast whatever you need for meal prepping. The best part about convection ovens is that they are evenly heated. You won't have some parts of your meal burnt while the other is still raw!

Microwave

To reheat your meals, a microwave is a must. This is what makes the meal prepping so great! Once you have prepped your meals, you stick it in the microwave for just a few minutes. Microwaves can be installed in your home or you can get a counter one for as little as $30.

Pressure Cooker

Today pressure cookers are becoming even more popular. They have been around for some time but nowadays there are electric pressure cookers which make cooking so much faster and convenient. Whether you have a traditional stovetop pressure cooker or an electric, it can make recipes a lot easier. It can cut down your cooking time by hours. Think shredded chicken in as little as 15 minutes! If you forget to put your meal in the slow cooker, your pressure cooker can usually take that frozen meal then cook it in under an hour. It also makes rice, beans, and other grains very quickly. This is highly recommended cooking equipment in your kitchen if you value time more than anything else. Instant Pot and Power Pressure Cooker XL are two popular choices in the market now.

Electric Lunch Box

If you want to keep your meals warm, an electric lunch box can help. Maybe you don't have a microwave at work or you just want it ready immediately at lunchtime! An electric lunch box can plug into your desk and warm up your food so it is ready by the time noon rolls around. Whether you are at an office or on the road, there are many different electric lunch boxes to choose from. Some plug into a standard wall plug but they also have ones that can plug into your car or plug into the USB port on your computer or laptop. Some electric lunch box models also come with a cooking function which means you can have your rice, porridge or even stews and soup cooked. Advanced features like an auto timer for cooking start/stop timing are also available for higher-end models.

Chapter 4   Food for Muscle Building

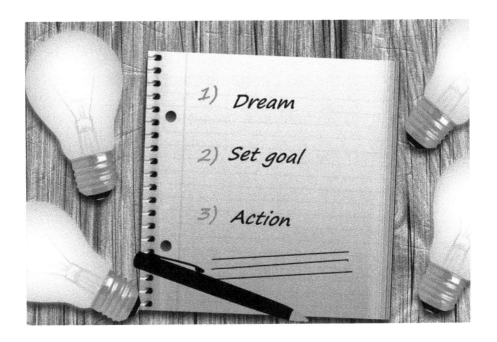

Working out is the hard part of being a bodybuilder. Eating is the easiest and most fun part. Still, there are many things to consider before putting food into your mouth. This chapter will focus on what foods to eat in order to help you gain your bodybuilder's body. You will get to know about the most popular foods that bodybuilders eat. You will also find out about 15 surprising foods you may have never thought to be great in building muscles.

The most common protein-rich foods can be found in your local market.\

- Egg white. If you don't like egg whites, then you shouldn't be a bodybuilder. Egg white is one of the best proteins you can find.

- Turkey and chicken breast

- Fish (especially tuna and salmon)

- Cheese

- Pork Chops

- Lean beef

- Tofu

- Soy beans

- Soymilk, yogurt and dairy milk.

- Nuts and some seeds like pumpkin seeds, peanuts, etc.

Just as it takes a bodybuilder a lot of discipline in the gym to do his workouts, it also take a lot of self-control to stick to a bodybuilder's diet composed of a balance of proteins and carbohydrates. Those that are strictly prohibited under this diet include those with refined sugars and artificial ingredients.

Protein-rich chicken and turkey are always available both in the local market and at grocery stores. More so are eggs. They are the most common yet the best muscle building foods you can eat for your meals. Those who might want to look for a little diversity in their diet can look for other sources of protein. Here's a surprise, these 15 foods can make your bodybuilding meals more interesting with their unexpected muscle building powers:

- Mackerel. This is from the tuna family but it packs higher levels of omega-3 content. Omega-3 assists in limiting recurrent inflammation resulting from intense muscle-training. Mackerel also has high levels of other nutrients needed by the body, such as zinc. This nutrient is needed to maintain the level of your testosterone.

- Beets. Nitrates are naturally found in beets. They improve your body's performance by increasing vasodilation. Studies show that eating 2 medium sized beets 1 ¼ hours before workouts improve body performance while reducing the level of exertion required to perform the exercises. They also decrease the amount of oxygen required to complete a workout.

- Greek Yogurt. Greek yogurt is produced by excess liquid and carbohydrates that were extracted from regular yogurt. The resulting compound has twice amount of protein. You have to take precautions though, because some companies manufacturing Greek yogurt products add thickeners to each product, lowering the pure Greek yogurt content.

- Sardines. While tuna is a very popular source of protein and other muscle building nutrients, sardines are even better. Canned sardines are very popular in the market just like tuna is and can be eaten straight out of the can. Four ounces of tuna may contain about 0.3 grams of omega-3 while the same amount of sardines may contain up to 1.8 grams of omega-3. As mentioned above, omega-3 reduces inflammation due to intense training, so adequate amount of this fat is needed by a bodybuilder. Older bodybuilders who may also have problems with anabolism deficits can turn to omega-3 for their problem.

- Kimchi. Kimchi is a traditional Korean food. This consists of fermented cabbage, onions, garlic, and other spices. Since kimchi is fermented, it contains good bacteria that help in digestion and absorption of nutrients.

- Chocolate milk. Protein powder may not be always available for you because of its cost. If this is the case, you can consume chocolate milk after your workout instead. Chocolate milk naturally has both of the fast and slow digesting protein. The chocolate in it gives an increase in the carbohydrate load of the drink. This gives more calories for muscle building and carbohydrates for a quicker recovery.

- Almonds. Compared to other nuts, almonds contain more protein and fiber. So instead of eating a lot of peanuts, try almonds instead.

- Vinegar. Nutrients should be brought to the muscle tissues and not the fat cells. This is the key to building a bodybuilder's lean muscles. And vinegar can help you with it. High-carbohydrate meals with vinegar in it cause more of the carbohydrates to be stored in muscle tissues.

- Avocado. Avocadoes are proven to have a unique and balanced combination of nutrients which makes it a great builder of muscles. At first, experts were skeptics about the fruit's muscle building power because of its high fat content, which may not be good for bodybuilders. But after some meticulous studies, scientists found out that avocadoes contain about 20 important nutrients and 250 calories. It also has 20 grams of fiber and 15 grams of monounsaturated fat. Avocadoes are also proven to help the body absorb antioxidants that can strengthen the immune system.

- Pea Protein. Pea protein can easily be digested. And unlike other vegetarian foods, they do not have compounds that hinder the absorption of nutrients. Also, pea protein has all essential amino acids at high levels, making it a great bodybuilder's food.

- Raspberries. Raspberries improve the function of the digestive system. Because of this, the body does better at absorbing nutrients gained from eaten foods.

- Kefir. Kefir is a fermented milk beverage. This contains probiotics and bioactive peptides allowing it to produce more muscle building nutrients. Each cup of kefir has more than 14 grams of protein.

- Lentils. Lentils are threefold in benefits. The most abundant nutrients in them are fiber, protein, and carbohydrates. Lentils come in three common varieties, all having a distinct color and flavor. If you are in a hurry to eat, red lentils are ideal foods as they can be prepared in just 15 minutes, compared to 30 to 45 minutes of other varieties.

- Broccoli. Some people would discourage you to eat broccoli because it can make you feel bloated fast. As a bodybuilder, you need a high calorie diet. Some people feel that the bloating results in early satiety, keeping the bodybuilder from getting the calories he needs. While this is true, broccoli is still a recommended muscle-building food as it helps reduce estrogen and gives a lot of antioxidants.

- Quinoa. Brown rice may be the bodybuilder's staple food, but quinoa provide a lot of unique advantages nutritionally and in other areas, compared to traditional carbohydrates. Although quinoa can be compared with a variety of rice, it is not really a grain. Quinoa plants can be compared to spinach. The unique aspect of quinoa is its muscle building properties. It contains amino acids that slow down the burning of calories, which gives a continuous infusion of energy through calories. Also, in practical terms, quinoa cooks faster than brown rice, making it a food for the bodybuilder on the rush.

Chapter 5   Tips for Building up Muscles

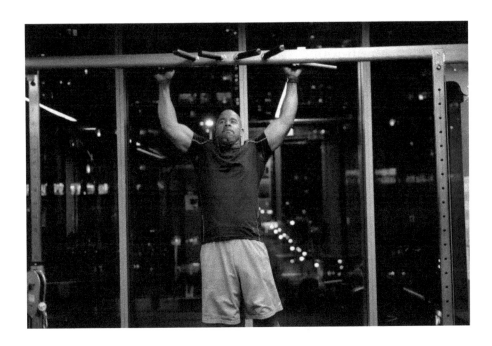

The biggest secret to building up muscle is to push your body into an anabolic state as quickly as you possibly can. While exercise is a clear requirement, it will only work if you use the right building blocks in the first place, and those building blocks come from the right nutritional approach. The following ten tips are the building blocks that you need to use to build up the maximum amount of muscle:

High-Calorie Intake is Vital

Most people see calories as the enemy and, although they may eat sufficient protein, they definitely do not consume anywhere near enough calories to put their body into an anabolic state. While the body needs protein to help it grow, it also needs the right intake of calories. One rule to work out your calorie count is to write down your bodyweight. Then multiply it by 10 if you are in good shape or by 12 if you are in excellent shape. Add between 1000 and 1500 to get your daily caloric intake. Many people advocate eating small meals on a regular basis throughout the day instead of eating just three meals. In this way, although your meals are smaller, they add up to a high enough intake of calories to push your body into that desired anabolic state in which your muscles will grow.

Eat Enough Carbohydrates

We all know that carbohydrates provide the fuel that our body burns, but more and more people are turning to low-carb diets. This forces the body to burn fat instead and, while this will give you the trim body you may desire, it will not give you the tools with which to build up those muscles. The exercises that you are doing require you to eat a high level of carbohydrates – the good ones – to enable your body to become saturated in glycogen. This means that protein levels are left alone and will never be used by the body to produce energy.

The higher the level of carbohydrates in your body, the more chances you have of remaining in an anabolic state. Moreover, carbs have a large part to play in how the body releases insulin, which is the single most powerful anabolic hormone that the body produces. The release of insulin goes on to promote adipocyte formation, protein synthesis, and gluconeogenesis.

Protein Consumption

As a rule of thumb, you need to eat between one and two grams for every pound that you weigh. So, if you weigh 200 lbs., you need to eat between 200 and 400 grams of protein every single day. That is a lot of protein to get through, and the easiest way to do it is to split your allowance up over several meals. This will help you to actually get through it all while also helping your body to absorb it better than if you ate vast amounts at one sitting. Do make sure that your protein comes from good foods, such as fish, beef, whey, chicken, and egg whites.

Eat Several Smaller Meals

So, your caloric intake is up to 4000, and that is a lot to face down. The best way to do this is to ditch your normal three meals a day and go for six or eight smaller ones instead. If you were to break 4000 calories up between six meals, each one would be about 600 calories, which is much more manageable.

If you are serious about adding muscle, making the switch to six bodybuilder-friendly meals a day is an absolute must. This creates a fuel reserve referred to as muscle glycogen, which promotes mass gain by energizing muscles and providing the fuel required for the muscles to heal. By supplying your body with nutrition six or more times per day, you give your muscles a constant supply of glycogen. If you only eat two of four meals a day, you deprive your muscles of this valuable fuel source. Furthermore, larger stores of glycogen increase water retention within muscles, thus encouraging growth and tissue repair.

Eating more frequently provides an almost non-stop supply of nutrients and protein. Muscles use amino acids, which are the building blocks of protein, to repair the damage caused by hard training. This causes muscles to grow larger by using amino acids to help manufacture the hormones that regulate growth and support the immune system. It is vital to have a strong immune system, as it plays a large role in recovering from a hard workout.

When planning your six meals, adopt the mantra of "eating clean." This means avoiding foods that do not contribute to muscle mass. These clean foods have more nutrients, are packed with vitamins, minerals, and fiber, and are prepared with very little or no added fat. Although fast food is definitely not considered clean food, if you are careful, you don't have to completely rule it out. If you have fast metabolism, you could eat fast food as one of your six meals on occasion and still have muscle gains as long as you follow certain restrictions and make sensible choices, like eating a burger without the mayonnaise or choosing a chicken sandwich with grilled instead of fried chicken and avoiding any breading. Skip out on the side orders, especially fries.

The first thing you will find is that your body doesn't like you eating these smaller meals, and it certainly isn't used to being fed six times a day! It will pay off though; you just have to stick at it. One more good reason for eating smaller meals more often is the insulin your body releases. When you eat, your blood sugar levels go up. To lower them again, your body will release insulin and, as you already know, insulin is a hormone required to keep your body in an anabolic state. The more insulin your body releases, the better it is, so eating smaller meals on a more regular basis will help with that.

Eat Plenty of Good Fat

If there is one mistake that many rookie bodybuilders make, it's that they don't eat enough good fat. For too long, we have been told to stay away from fat, but good fats are highly beneficial and are actually required by your body. There is also a direct link between good fat and testosterone levels. Without sufficient good fats in your diet, your muscles cannot possibly grow.

Eat a Good Meal Before a Workout

Bodybuilding workouts are hard work, and your body needs sufficient fuel to keep going. The best foods to eat before your work out are slow-burning carbs, such as rice and pasta. The reason you should eat this is because they take much longer before they convert to glucose. This means that your blood sugar levels stay consistent for longer, providing you with the energy needed for the workout and stopping energy crashes. Make sure you include a decent serving of protein with the meal.

Eat a Good Meal After a Workout

In the same way that you need a decent meal before, you also need to make sure you have a good meal after your workout. The only difference is that this meal needs to contain a high level of protein and the fast-burning carbs, as opposed to the slow burners. The best thing would be a good protein shake and sugar in one form or another.

When you work out, your body is in a catabolic state, and that needs to be destroyed so that it can grow back much stronger and bigger than before. However, if you don't give your body the right building blocks, it can't possibly repair itself efficiently. The average person would benefit from a protein shake with about 40 g to 75 g of carbohydrates. Don't wait though – drink the shake the minute you finish training.

Drink Sufficient Water

Hydration is important to all of us, bodybuilder or otherwise. Most people do not consume enough water while they are exercising, which is really counterproductive when you consider that the body is made up of 70% water. Dehydration has a detrimental effect on the size of your muscles – it is thought that just one pound of muscle can hold up to three pounds of water. Add that up, and it comes to quite a bit of size!

Use Good-quality Supplements

Many supplements are cheap, but these are not the ones you want. If your pocket can accommodate it, use proper high-quality supplements, such as creatine, protein powders, joint formula, glutamine, and multivitamins. The simple reason is that these supplements work for as long as you do.

Get Enough Rest

In their bid to build a good body, many rookies make the mistake of thinking that they have to work out and stay on the go as often as possible. The one thing they forget about – and perhaps the most important thing – is rest. Your muscles will not grow, and they will not repair themselves properly if you don't rest. The way it works is that when you work out, you "break" your body by giving it the stimulus it needs to get growing. In order to be put back together again, your body needs the correct combination of nutrients and sufficient rest. Try to rest up for at least two days of the week, and keep in mind that rest means rest and nothing else.

Characteristics of a Good Nutrition Plan for Bodybuilding

Making a meal plan is not always easy. There are things to consider for you to achieve your bodybuilding goals fully. This chapter will teach you the characteristics of a good nutrition program for bodybuilding. Without further ado, here are the key qualities of a proper muscle-bulking meal plan:

1. It should focus on small meals and portions rather than large ones. Your metabolism increases when you eat small meals frequently rather than eat one large meal per day. Increased metabolism results in an increase in the capability to burn more fat. It is advisable that you eat four to six meals a day, with intervals of two to three hours.

2. Meals should contain protein, carbohydrates, and fats. To achieve the desired results, you must observe a balanced diet with the correct ratio of these three nutrients. The correct ratio, as science suggests, is 40% protein, 40% carbohydrates, and 20% fats.

3. Your nutrition program should be compatible with the other aspects of your life. It must contain meal plans that suit your lifestyle and are applicable for a long period of time. Necessary changes should only be minimal. Moreover, it would be difficult for you to adapt to a new nutrition plan every couple of weeks. It is important that you are consistent so that you will achieve your desired goals.

4. Your meal plan should be designed in accordance with your bodybuilding goals. In other words, you must

first specify your bodybuilding goals before you begin creating a meal plan. How much muscle do you want to grow? Which part of your body would you like to become more muscular? This is important to note because there are meal plans especially designed to achieve particular results.

5. Meal ingredients should be accessible. There are meal plans with dishes that are so complicated that you would no longer know where to find the ingredients. Make sure that when you design your meal plan, the ingredients are simple yet healthy. Remember that your nutrition plan should be applicable for the rest of your life, which is why it is important that you have easy access to the ingredients.

Now that you know the characteristics of a good meal plan, the next step is to create your own. The succeeding chapters will share sample meal plans that you could use for five days.

Chapter 6   A 12-Week Guide to Bodybuilding

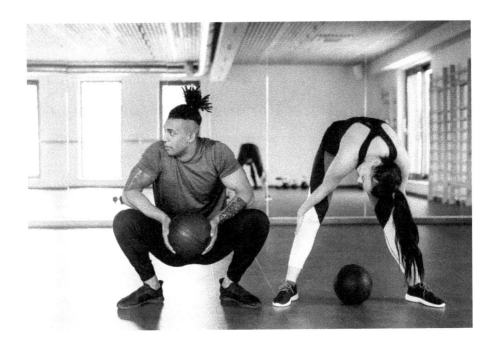

You have already learned about the diet that you need to have if you want to grow bigger muscles. Protein is necessary, along with other nutrients. You can get the nutrients that you need from food, but you can also get them from supplements. Keep in mind that supplements cannot be taken alone. You still have to eat properly. Supplements are only meant to improve your diet and ensure that you get all the nutrients that your body needs.

Anyway, here are the supplements that you can take in order to help you grow bigger muscles:

Chromium. It is a mineral that aids the body in dealing with carbohydrate consumption.

Vitamin C. It is inexpensive and can be easily obtained. It is also the ultimate antioxidant. If you lack in this vitamin, you can be more prone to colds. You need vitamin C to improve your immune system. Ideally, you should take at least three grams per day.

Multivitamin. Experts recommend taking one to two multivitamins per day to ensure that you get all the vitamins you need.

- Whey protein. It is easy to prepare and nutritious. It is also low in fat and quick to digest. You can take it to work. Forty grams of whey protein is equivalent to a few ounces of turkey or steak.

Sample Menu Plan 1

Meal 1	Fat	Protein	Carbohydrates	Calories
7 egg whites	0	21	0	105
1 cup of oatmeal	6	10	54	300
1 banana	0	12	30	125
Total	6	43	84	530

Meal 2	Fat	Protein	Carbohydrates	Calories
4 oz. of chicken breast	2	26	0	122
1 cup of brown rice	1	6	7	209
½ cup of vegetables	0	2	7	36
Total	3	34	51	367

Meal 3	Fat	Protein	Carbohydrates	Calories
4 oz. of turkey	4	20	2	121
2 pieces of bread	1	5	31	183
Total	5	25	33	304

Meal 4	Fat	Protein	Carbohydrates	Calories
4 oz. of steak	6	26	0	173
6 oz. of baked sweet potato	0	3	42	180
½ cup of steamed broccoli	0	3	10	56
Total	6	33	52	409

Meal 5	Fat	Protein	Carbohydrates	Calories
4 oz. of chicken breast	2	26	0	122
2 tbsp. Efa's	22	0	0	200
3/4 cup of steamed spinach	0	1	6	28
Total	24	27	6	350

Daily Totals	Fat	Protein	Carbohydrates	Calories
Nutrient grams	68	191	235	2,310

Recommended Foods:

Protein:

Turkey breast

Chicken breast

Ground turkey

Salmon

Swordfish

Crab

Tuna

Shrimp

Lobster

Lean steaks

Lean ham

Low-fat cottage cheese

Soy protein

Whey protein

Protein powders

Egg white

Carbohydrates:

Sweet potatoes

Leafy green vegetables

Yams

Pumpkin

Squash

Brown rice

Oatmeal

Pasta

Beans

Barley

Whole wheat bread

Sample Menu Plan 2

This menu plan is much easier to prepare. Every one of these meals contains about four hundred calories. They also have higher protein content than the previous sample menu plan. For every one hundred and ninety pound-man, it is about one and a half grams per pound of bodyweight.

Meal 1 (8:00 AM)
1 cup of oatmeal
1 sweet potato
2 scoops of whey protein combined with skim milk

Meal 2 (10:30 AM)
1 cup of oatmeal
Cottage cheese

Workout period (12:00 – 1:00 PM)

Meal 4 (3:00 PM)
Salad
2 wheat bread
4 to 6 oz. of lean turkey

Meal 5 (6:15 PM)
Salad
8 oz. of salmon
200 calories Efa's

Meal 6 (7:30 PM)
Salad
Chicken breast
200 calories Efa's

Key points of this diet:

Never starve yourself.

Reduce your calories gradually. You can decrease two hundred and fifty every week.

Spread out your calories evenly by eating five to six meals per day.

Drink plenty of water and cut back on beverages high in sugar.

Be consistent with your diet.

- Keep in mind that this is a twelve-week program. So, you should not rush. Do not try to do everything all at once. It is a scientifically proven diet, so there is nothing for you to worry about. All you have to do is follow the meal plan and you would be fine.

Master Meal Plan During Non-Workout Days

When it comes to building muscles, you have to follow a specific meal plan during your workout days. Similarly, you have to follow a specific meal plan during your non-workout days in order to maintain consistency. Here is a sample menu plan you can follow during your rest days.

Meal 1	
No. of carbohydrates	75 grams
No. of protein	35 grams
No. of fats	15 grams
No. of kilocalories	575 kcals
No. of servings of meat	4
No. of servings of fat	3
No. of servings of fruit	1
No. of servings of carbohydrates	3
No. of servings of milk	1

Meal 2	
No. of carbohydrates	60 grams
No. of protein	35 grams
No. of fats	20 grams
No. of kilocalories	560 kcals
No. of servings of meat	5

No. of servings of fat	4
No. of servings of fruit	1
No. of servings of carbohydrates	3
No. of servings of milk	0
Meal 3	
No. of carbohydrates	50 grams
No. of protein	35 grams
No. of fats	15 grams
No. of kilocalories	475 kcals
No. of servings of meat	5
No. of servings of fat	3
No. of servings of fruit	1
No. of servings of carbohydrates	3
No. of servings of milk	0

Meal 4	
No. of carbohydrates	50 grams
No. of protein	35 grams
No. of fats	15 grams
No. of kilocalories	475 kcals
No. of servings of meat	4
No. of servings of fat	3
No. of servings of fruit	1
No. of servings of carbohydrates	2

No. of servings of milk	1

Meal 5	
No. of carbohydrates	40 grams
No. of protein	42 grams
No. of fats	15 grams
No. of kilocalories	463 kcals
No. of servings of meat	6
No. of servings of fat	3
No. of servings of fruit	2
No. of servings of carbohydrates	2
No. of servings of milk	0

Meal 6	
No. of carbohydrates	10 grams
No. of protein	35 grams
No. of fats	15 grams
No. of kilocalories	315 kcals
No. of servings of meat	5
No. of servings of fat	3
No. of servings of fruit	2
No. of servings of carbohydrates	0
No. of servings of milk	0

Total carbohydrates	285 grams
Total fat	95 grams
Total protein	217 grams
Total calories	2863 grams

Here is a suggested meal plan for the days that you do not work out:

Meal 1		
268 grams of egg whites	113.4 grams of lean turkey breast	228 grams of non-fat cottage cheese
25.8 grams of almonds	31.8 grams of peanut butter or almond butter	85 grams of avocado
18 grams of raisins	184 grams of grapefruit	64 grams of banana
60 grams of dry oatmeal	99 grams of whole grain muffin	96 grams of whole grain bread
170 grams of light yogurt	237 milliliters of non-fat milk	170 grams of plain non-fat yogurt

Meal 2		

41.75 grams of canned tuna in water	41.75 grams of grilled tilapia	41.7 grams of grilled chicken breast
34.4 grams of almonds	42.4 grams of peanut butter or almond butter	113.4 grams of avocado
92 grams of apple	85 grams of pear	99 grams of peeled orange
60 grams of dry oatmeal	171 grams of baked sweet potatoes	93 grams of cooked brown rice

Meal 3		
41.75 grams of grilled chicken breast	41.75 grams of grilled tilapia	285 grams of non-fat cottage cheese
25.8 grams of almonds	13.5 grams of olive oil	85 grams of avocado
78 grams of steamed broccoli	62.5 grams of steamed green beans	125 grams of steamed spinach
93 grams of cooked brown rice	171 grams of baked sweet potatoes	138 grams of whole grain pasta

Meal 4		
40 grams of whey protein	113.4 grams of grilled tilapia	113.4 grams of grilled chicken breast
28 grams of peanuts	31.8 grams of peanut butter or almond butter	85 grams of avocado
78 grams of steamed broccoli	62.5 grams of steamed green beans	113 grams of steamed asparagus
129 grams of cooked brown rice	114 grams of baked sweet potatoes	33.4 grams of cream of wheat
28.35 grams of light yogurt	237 milliliters of non-fat milk	170 grams of plain non-fat yogurt

Meal 5		
170.1 grams of grilled tilapia	170.1 grams of grilled lean fillet	170.1 grams of grilled chicken breast
22.5 grams of walnuts	13.5 grams of olive oil	85 grams of avocado

330 grams of lettuce	125 grams of steamed green beans	226 grams of steamed asparagus
180 grams of tomato		
128.7 grams of cooked brown rice	114 grams of baked yams	92 grams of whole grain pasta

Meal 6		
50 grams of whey protein	285 grams of non-fat cottage cheese	41.75 grams of grilled chicken breast
25.8 grams of almonds	31.8 grams of peanut butter or almond butter	85 grams of avocado
156 grams of steamed broccoli	125 grams of steamed green beans	226 grams of steamed asparagus

Chapter 7   Freezer Meals

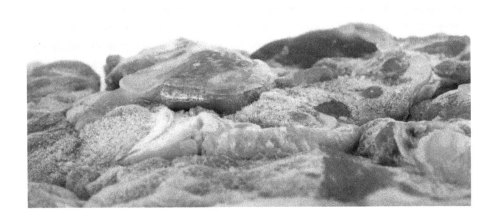

When things get really busy and you are struggling to prepare your meals, freezer meals can help. You can make freezer meals part of your weekly meal prepping or you can make them up to a month in advance. They are wonderful for ensuring that you have delicious homemade meals ready to go on those nights when you just don't have time to cook or just don't feel like it and they are a great way to make sure you stick to your diet.

Bulk cooking is something that many people have started doing in their lives in order to reduce the amount of time that they spend in the kitchen after a long day at work. Creating freezer meals does take some time, however, it is entirely possible to create healthy freezer meals that you can have for dinner every night while prepping your fresh breakfasts, lunches, and snacks.

Freezer meals have many benefits, including saving money on those expensive takeout meals when you just don't feel like cooking, but it is going to give you more freedom from being chained to your kitchen every night. Pulling a bag out of the freezer and dumping it in the crockpot before you leave for work, or grabbing a casserole out of the freezer when you get home will give you time to focus on more important things. Of course, this is also going to help ensure that your kitchen stays cleaner as well.

Freezer meals are going to allow you to enjoy some down time, they can be taken with you when you go on vacation, and you always know exactly what is in the food that you are preparing so if there are any allergies in the family, you don't have to worry.

What Can Be Frozen?

You can freeze stews, casseroles, soups, pasta sauces, chicken, burritos, chili, and so many other meals. This means that you don't just have to eat foods that can be made in a crockpot every night. It is very easy to bag up vegetables for fajitas or stir fries, and you can even create meal kits.

Desserts from the freezer are wonderful as well. There is nothing better than being able to pull out a fresh apple pie and bake it whenever the urge hits. You can stock up on healthy fruits when they are in season and at their lowest price then create amazing desserts with them.

How Does It Work?

Freezer meals are prepared ahead of time, which makes them a great addition to your meal prep routine. You can create freezer meals a few different ways. You can make them on the day that you work on your meal prep and make a week to a month's worth of freezer meals. Or the other option is to simply double or even quadruple your meals as you cook them and then place the extra servings in your freezer. What you choose will depend completely upon how much time you have to spare and how many meals you want to create.

What is really great about freezer meals is that you are able to purchase all of the items that you need in one shopping trip which is going to save you a ton of money as well as a ton of time, especially if you create freezer meals for the entire month.

Freezer Meal Tips

1. Make sure that you schedule enough time. It is going to take about 1 hour to make 16 freezer meals. This will usually be 4 recipes made 4 times. Therefore, if you want to make an entire months' worth of freezer meals, you will want to make sure you plan for about 2 hours of cooking.

2. To reduce the amount of time that you are spending on your freezer meals, you can keep chopped vegetables such as onions or peppers as well as cooked meat and cheese on hand.

3. If you want to reduce the amount that you are spending on groceries, make sure that you stock up on soups, canned tomatoes, meats, sauces, and beans when they are on sale.

4. Make sure that you are using a freezer bag that is of high quality. You do not want to purchase the cheapest freezer bags possible when you are making freezer meals because you want your foods to be protected.

5. When you freeze your meals, lay the bag on the side so that it flattens out, after the meals are frozen, you can move them to create more space.

6. Thaw your freezer meals out in a large bowl in your fridge in order to ensure the bags do not leak. Freezer bags can get holes in them and they will at some point. Putting the freezer bag in a bowl to thaw ensures not only that you do not have a huge mess in your fridge, but that you do not lose any of your food as well.

7. When you are creating freezer meals, use freezer bags instead of storage containers. Not only is this going to take up less space, but it is going to ensure that there is less for you to clean up.

8. Place your freezer bags in a storage container when you are filling them up to prevent them from spilling.

9. When you are creating multiples of the same recipe, line the bags up and measure out each of the ingredients into the bags once. For example, place all of the onions into each of the freezer bags when creating chili, followed by all of the canned tomatoes and so on.

10. Always make sure that you are labeling all of the freezer bags with the recipe that they contain, cooking directions, as well as the date that they were made.

11. Start out using recipes that are specifically for freezer meals. You will find some of these at the end of this book. Recipes that are written for freezer meals are going to walk you through the process step by step.

12. Always make sure that you are planning out the freezer meal process. You will need to plan

time to decide what meals you are going to make, to plan your shopping trips and your prepping days. You want to make sure that you know what stores you will be going to, what coupons you will be using if any, and even what order you will visit the stores in. The better planned the day, the more successful you are going to be.

Choose a variety of meals that are going to require very little prep work and that have overlapping ingredients. Choosing recipes with overlapping ingredients is going to reduce your amount of prep time.

14.   Always make one batch of a recipe and try it before making it in bulk. You do not want to end up with several meals that you do not like or no one will eat.

15.   Do as much of the prep work as you can at the same time. For example, I begin by prepping all of my vegetables, then I focus on cooking all of the meats. While the meats cook, I open all of the cans of tomatoes, sauces, and so on then pour them into my bags. By the time that the meat is done and cooled, all I have to do is put it in the bags and zip them up.

16. Freezer meals will keep for up to 3 months, so it is important for you to keep the freezer organized and keep a running list of what meals you have prepared. This will ensure nothing goes to waste and you know what your options are when you want to use them.

17. Make sure that you let the freezer meal cool to room temperature before you freeze it. This usually only takes about 30 minutes.

18. Remove as much of the air from the freezer bags as you can before you freeze them. If you are preparing foods in a baking dish, cover them with plastic wrap and then foil in order to keep the air out and ensure they do not get freezer burnt.

19. Muffins and breads freeze really well. You will want to wrap each muffin or slice of bread individually, which will also help with portion control.

20. If you want to freeze individual portions for smaller meals such as lunch, you can use silicone muffin tins. Simply freeze the soup, stew or other food in the muffin tin and then pop them out and place them all in a freezer bag. When you are ready to eat, just pull out one serving.

Foods That Do Not Freeze Well

1. Potatoes. When you freeze potatoes, it changes the texture as well as the taste. While freezing them will prevent them from spoiling, it is likely that you are not going to want to eat them after they have thawed. However, mashed potatoes are fine for freezing.

2. Vegetables and fruits that have a high water content or are delicate such as watermelon, citrus fruit, tomatoes, and cucumbers. It is possible for you to freeze some of these foods, for example, tomatoes, if they are going to be cooked but do not expect them to come out of the freezer the same way that you put them in.

3. Any sauce or gravy that you have used cornstarch to thicken is not going to freeze

well because they tend to separate as well as break down in the freezer. Instead of freezing the gravy, simply freeze the stock, and then add the cornstarch after it has been reheated.

4. Egg whites will become rubbery if you freeze them as will celery. If you are freezing a recipe that contains either, make sure that you chop them finely before freezing.

5. Mayonnaise is going to break down if it is put in the freezer. If you are freezing a recipe that needs mayonnaise, leave the mayonnaise out and add it in last, when you are ready to cook it.

6. If you are making cakes for desserts, you will want to make sure that you are using a butter cream frosting on them. Other frostings do not freeze well.

7. Pastas tend to become too soft if they are frozen and reheated. Personally, I prefer to cook the pasta fresh, 8 to 12 minutes of boiling pasta in order to have a delicious dinner is fine with me. If you want to do it this way, simply add all of the ingredients into your freezer bag except the pasta, then cook the pasta when you are ready to eat the meal.

If you want the pasta pre-cooked, under-cook the pasta before putting it in your freezer bag.

8. Cheeses are fine to freeze; however, yogurt and sour cream will separate when you freeze them.

Preparing For Freezer Meal Prep

Once you decide that you are going to use freezer meals as part of your meal prep routine, you will probably find yourself wondering exactly how you can do it. While having a freezer full of meals that are ready to do is wonderful and makes your life a lot easier, it can seem a bit overwhelming at first. However, if you follow these directions, it does not have to be.

1. Take inventory of what you already have. This is one thing that so many people forget to do before they start planning their meals which leads to being overrun with cans of tomatoes or beans. While having extra food on hand is not a bad thing, if saving money is a priority, there is no reason for you to not use up the food that you have.

The idea is to not have much of anything left in your cabinets after your meal prep is done except for some baking staples, spices, grains, and maybe some pasta.

Make a list of everything that you have in your cabinets as well as your fridge and start thinking about how you can use that food up. Perhaps you have a few squash left in the fridge and a bag of sweet potatoes. You can easily roast these and toss them in with your lunch. If you have beans in your cabinet, consider making a chili or four and freezing them to eat later.

2. Check your sales fliers. Let's face it, no matter how much money we have, no one wants to overspend on groceries when we know we could use the money elsewhere. This means that before you start planning those freezer meals, you will want to grab the sales flyers from the stores that you shop at (or look them up online) and figure out what is on sale and how you can use it. For example, if you find chicken on sale for 99 cents a pound, try to plan a lot of your meals around that sale.

3. Think about your needs. Do you need easy meals that are not going to take a long time to prep or can you devote your entire day to meal prep? Maybe you want to prep simple breakfasts and lunches but want more complex dinners. However, you choose to create your meals you need to do so with your

needs in mind. You do not want to choose a bunch of crockpot freezer meals if you know the food is not going to make it into the crockpot in the mornings.

4. The next step is to start making a list of all of the ingredients that you are going to need. Divide your list according to what store you will purchase the items at and what aisle if possible. For example, I will purchase my produce and almond milk at one store, then my tofu and a few other items are purchased at another store, and I even go to a third store. If I did not separate my list into what specific store I was going to get each item, my shopping day could become very stressful and I could forget to purchase a lot of my ingredients.

Go through your list twice to make sure that you have included everything that you need. I find it easiest if I create a list with every ingredient that I need. I will start with my recipes and write down what I need, doubling or tripling depending on how many freezer meals I plan on making. After I have a list of every ingredient, I will condense it down, for example, if I need 3 bags of brown rice for one recipe and 2 for another, I just add them together and write down 5 bags of brown rice. As I am doing this, I will have three sheets of paper.

Each sheet of paper is going to be for one specific store. As I go through the ingredients, I will write what I need down on the paper for the store that I plan on purchasing it at. Then, I will go through the list a second time making sure that you have not forgotten to add anything to your list.

> 5. After you have created your list, it is time for you to go shopping. There are times that just thinking about shopping can wear a person out but if this happens, just remind yourself that when you are done prepping your meals, you and your family are going to eat better for the entire month.

When you go shopping, try to go alone, if you take your children you could become distracted and you could end up purchasing items that you do not really need. It is a terrible thing when you have all of your food cooking and suddenly you realize that you did not purchase an item that was on your list because you were distracted.

> 6. Finally, after you have done your shopping it is time for you to prep your meals.

When you are first starting out, I would suggest that you only focus on one week's worth of food. It is very easy for you to prep your breakfast, lunch, and snacks using the method discussed, and it is very easy to create a week's worth of dinners using freezer meals.

It is likely that while you are creating your week's worth of freezer meals, you will realize how simple it would be to create multiple meals and eventually you will be able to do this.

When you make a month's worth of freezer meals, not only are you going to free up a ton of your time in the evenings, but you are also going to reduce the amount of time that you spend prepping your meals each week because you will only have to worry about breakfast, lunch, and snacks.

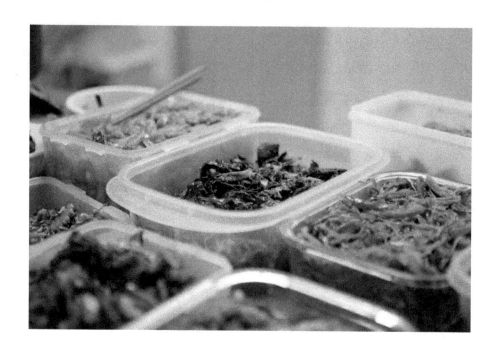

Freezer Meal Benefits

1. Making large batches of food and separating them out into freezer bags to use over a long period of time is going to save you time, money, and energy. When you know that you have meals that are ready to eat right at your fingertips, you are going to be less tempted to go out to eat, cleaning up after dinner is going to be a breeze and you can create freezer meals in the same time that it would take to make one meal.

2. You are able to cook once and eat many times. When I make my freezer meals, I will make four of each of the seven dinners, which means that I can cook once and eat for an entire month.

3. You are able to enjoy healthy home-cooked meals with minimal stress. Of course, prep day can be a bit stressful for anyone, however, if you plan it out properly and allow yourself plenty of time for your planning and prepping it does not have to be stressful at all. In fact, meal prepping can be one of the most relaxing times of your week.

4. One of the things that most people love about having freezer meals is that they always know what they are going to have for dinner. They do not find themselves sitting at their desk 30 minutes before it is time to go home wondering what they are going to cook. Nor do they find themselves standing in front of a fridge looking at the food that they have but still unable to come up with any ideas.

Freezer meals and meal prepping help to reduce the stress in your life as well as the anxiety. It saves you time as well as money and it ensures that you will always know what is going into the food that you are eating and when you come home from work at night, you are going to be able to relax instead of standing over a stove and cooking for an hour then cleaning up.

Chapter 8 What Are Macros And How Do They Count

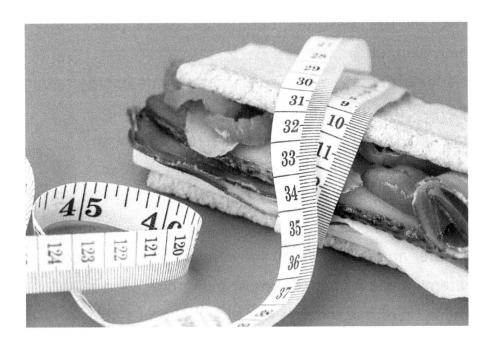

The macronutrients that constitute our diet are:

The Carbohydrates: also called carbon carbohydrates, sugars or more commonly, are the primary source of energy. They also contain the fibers, which we will define a little later.

The Fat: fatty acids also called "fat" or fat are molecules that form the organic fat. They play an important role in the constitution of cell membranes, energy production, and body temperature and more generally in the metabolism of the human being.

The Proteins: they are essential molecules for the life of cells and the constitution of human tissues (muscles, hair, skin, etc.).

Macronutrients are molecules that provide energy to our body or that participate directly or indirectly in metabolism. They are called "macro" in order to differentiate them from micronutrients such as vitamins, minerals, enzymes, etc.

They are called macros because we need them in greater amounts than micronutrients, which include vitamins and minerals. Almost everything we eat is made up of macronutrients, and sometimes also micronutrients, which we need in smaller quantities.

Carbohydrates

It is the main source of energy of the body.

As you have guessed, it's about sugars, and yes sugars, we'll always need them. Everything depends then which sugars to privilege, and there, it becomes more complicated.

In theory, these are the complex sugars to favor at the expense of simple sugars, but that does not help you much!

What are the foods based on complex sugars and those based on simple sugars?

Simple sugars have a high glycemic index (Glucose and sucrose ...) they are present in sweets, pastries, classic white sugar, in many prepared dishes, sauces (ketchup, bbq sauce, sweet and sour)

Complex sugars, meanwhile, have a low glycemic index; they are present in cereals (whole grains, attention!) and legumes.

Sugar in fruits is also an excellent source of energy, but we must not forget that fructose must first be treated in the liver before 'be used by the body, and it cannot be part of the complex sugars, it is a so-called fast sugar, but does not have a too high glycemic index, (IG: 20 against 100 for glucose), which differentiates it especially glucose classic is that the carbohydrate intake is supplemented with a contribution of fiber, minerals and vitamins.

THE PROTIDES

In common parlance we often tend to call them "proteins", but this is an abuse of language, and yes, in fact the protides is a sort of "family" grouping proteins, amino acids, and peptides.

When we talk about proteins "protiderotides" we immediately think of our muscles, and yes you know well they are made up, but we must not forget that they are also made of 70% water, moreover the water content of our body represents on average about 65% of our mass, small parenthesis

Back to our proteins, except the muscles (myosin, actin, myoglobin) , they are also present in our hair, nail our skin (keratin), but also in our red blood cells (globin). They provide a multitude of functions within the cells:

- Cell renewal
- Role of protection (hair, nails, skin)
- Physiological functioning (information transmission, digestion, immune defense)
- Secondary energy role (after carbohydrates)
- and it is also our only source of nitrogen (essential for life) , and yes it is a present element to link amino acids to each other.
- Proteins are of animal or vegetable origin (legumes, cereals)

Contrary to many received ideas, vegetable proteins are not of less good quality than animal proteins, on the contrary.

Indeed, animal proteins also contain so-called saturated fats (we'll talk about it later), favoring weight gain, cardiovascular risks and clot formation, on the contrary vegetable proteins are rich in fibers without any saturated fat.

LIPIDS

Despite their demonization, it is a primordial macro nutrient essential to our proper functioning.

Lipids are an important energy store, they are essential to regulate the temperature of our body, and very importantly, they are one of the major constituents of membranes   and the nervous system, indeed lipids surround and strengthen our lymph.

On the other hand, lipids are not all of the same quality! This is where the difference, always and again, good and bad fats, so we distinguish different types of fatty acids: saturated, monounsaturated or polyunsaturated.

The saturated = to limit! They increase the cardiovascular risk as stated above (contained in fatty meats, sausages, butter or cream, vegetable fats biscuits and industrial dishes)

Mono-unsaturated = also called omega-9 contained in oilseeds (almonds, hazelnuts, walnuts ...) and avocado

Poly-unsaturated = these are omega 6 and 3, these are essential fatty acids, our body is unable to synthesize them, they contribute to the proper functioning of our cardiovascular system, some studies have demonstrated that omega-3 fatty acids promote lipolysis (provision of fat to provide energy to the body) it is not beautiful, so do not hesitate to consume virgin oils first cold pressed (olive oil, rapeseed),also in oily fish, but I cannot encourage you to consume since they too often contain heavy metals such as mercury, and especially for our biodiversity and ethics, it is better to leave them there where he is, it was the little ethical parenthesis

An individual's macros are calculated as a percentage of the total calories consumed. "So, for example, if you are an active middle-aged and 60k-weight individual who goes to the gym regularly and follow a 1600-calorie diet, you need 40% of your calories to come from carbohydrates, 30% of proteins and 30% of fats. These proportions would be normal for those who do not train for a living, or for people who are active, but not for endurance athletes. This is what those calculations would look like:

1600 x 0.40 = 640 calories from carbohydrates

1600 x 0.30 = 480 calories of protein

1600 x 0.30 = 480 calories from fat

"To convert those calories figures into grams, carbohydrates and proteins are divided by 4, because both carbohydrates and proteins provide 4 calories per

gram, "and fat by 9, because fat contributes 9 calories.
per gram. " This is how those calculations would work:

640/4 = 160 grams of carbohydrates

480/4 = 120 grams of protein

480/9 = 53 grams of fat

The proportion of macros will change according to your objectives. "It is important to take into account your level of activity and the type of exercises you do,
For example, if you are strength training you will need to increase your protein intake to facilitate muscle recovery and prevent injuries. While if you focus more on cardio, you will have to increase carbohydrates to prevent the wear of glycogen stores.

WHAT IS THE EASIEST WAY TO CALCULATE YOUR OWN MACROS?

When entering your data in an online macro calculator: age, height, weight, sex, activity level, target weight, frequency and intensity with which you lift weights. If It Fits Your Macros, which also asks when you want to achieve your goals, or Healthy Eater , which is simpler, but produces similar calculations.

The Benefits Of Counting Macros

A positive aspect of eating by adjusting to your macros is that each macro performs a unique function. As runners or endurance athletes, it is important to have enough carbohydrates to avoid "crashing into the wall", but you also don't have to be too forgiving.

It's about getting the right amount of each one right, so as not to fall short or exceed your body's needs. By achieving that balance, your body will function at its highest level and you will recover properly. It also activates other systems such as immune, digestive and sleep. "It's like a group of workers in which everyone does their job so that the whole body works at its maximum performance.

It is clear that this "work" depends on your level of activity and your objectives. "If you are an athlete, macros are very important. Also, if you eat adjusting to your macros, you don't have to eliminate any important food groups or deprive yourself of anything.

But if you want to lose fat, gain muscle, it is very important to consider the source and quality of the food you eat. "I have seen people who count macros stuffing themselves with donuts because 'it fits their macros', but they perform less and feel worse than if they had opted for sweet potatoes or other types of carbohydrates," he adds.

THE BAD THING ABOUT COUNTING MACROS

In an IIFYM diet, the important thing is not to deprive yourself of something, but to feed you so that your body functions in the most effective way. But counting macros can take time. Not only do you have to know the proportions, but you also have to measure food on an appropriate scale. So if you feel lazy to weigh everything you eat, counting macros is not made for you.

In addition, monitoring, tracking and weighing everything you eat can create an unhealthy relationship with food. Anytime the numbers go up and you like to control your diet. But if you have suffered eating disorders in the past, counting macros is probably not a good idea.

Like any other diet, counting macros is not a panacea. It can help you make the body function very effectively, and even serve you to reach certain goals, but remember that the most important thing is the quality of what you eat. As an athlete, you know that diet is only part of the equation, so the best is what best suits your lifestyle and, therefore, you manage to maintain in the long term.

Tips For A Healthy Life Through Meal Plan

- Write your goals in our quadrant and with the tests in a visible place, Start with a simple exercise routine, for example going for a walk
- Eliminate sources of liquid calories, coffee, soda, alcohol, replace them with water, green tea and natural juices
- Template to write what you eat (without forgetting anything)
- Make your exercise day increasing the time and intensity of them
- Change from 3 large meals to 6 small ones, each day adding fruit, vegetables and protein at all meals
- Make a shopping list with healthy foods and go shopping with a full stomach, with a satiated appetite
- Weigh yourself and write on a table as you move forward in your challenge
- Choose an activity to do 3 times a week, it can be a sport, a dance class or just keep walking longer or with more intensity
- Always plan the next week's menu

- Add more fruit and vegetables to your diet than you have ever eaten before or long ago you eliminated from the diet
- Make sure you are drinking enough water, about 8 glasses (2 liters of water per day approx)
- Pay attention to the amount of fiber you consume per day, at least 35gr is recommended, if you do not reach this figure, consume some almonds (these will also help you control your appetite)

All About Hygiene

There are no harmful substances are not involved in food but nobody has to take unnecessary risks. A few important hygiene principles usually provide sufficient protection.

Wash & clean

Pesticides are used for pest control. To remove them from fruits and vegetables, a short rinse with water is not enough. Apples, tomatoes and co. Must be thoroughly rinsed under lukewarm water - preferably with a soft brush.

Afterwards, you should dry solid fruits and vegetables with a cloth. Organic farming largely dispenses with the use of pesticides. Therefore, organic products often less burdened. Nevertheless, also here: wash thoroughly before consumption. Many heavy metals can be eliminated as well.

For salads - especially from conventional outdoor cultivation - you should always remove the outer leaves, as attach here particularly many pesticides. In fruits and vegetables that grows or is sold on busy roads, can also adhere pollutants from exhaust gases, brake pad and tire abrasion. Again, wash thoroughly, peel fruits and vegetables if necessary.

Tip: Use a different board and knife to cut and process raw meat than for the rest of the meal. Anyone who cuts peppers and lettuce with a knife with which he has previously cut chicken breasts can carry salmonella into the lettuce. Meat and fish are often contaminated with bacteria, which die only when cooking or roasting.

COOL WELL

Food infections are common. Mostly it is due to a lack of hygiene. Eggs are particularly vulnerable. Salmonella can also occur on and in the meat. To prevent salmonella from multiplying too much, these foods are in the fridge: eggs in the door and meat and fish and raw sausage as far down as possible, but above the vegetable compartments - where it is the coldest.

When cooking or frying: High temperatures (from 80 degrees Celsius) kill the germs. However, eggs or meat must be heated for a sufficient amount of time.

Tip: To avoid salmonella in the food.

CAREFULLY FRY

Benzpyrene, so-called polycyclic aromatic hydrocarbons (PAHs) are highly carcinogenic. They are produced by frying, baking, grilling and smoking. But they also occur in car exhaust and cigarette smoke. This is especially the case with the smoking of fish and meat.

Whether smoking, roasting or baking: the higher the temperatures, the more PAHs are produced. Therefore always cut off black, burnt places on meat and baked goods generously. Fry with high temperatures to kill germs, but it does not have to be too strong. The Federal Office for Risk Assessment recommends a core temperature in the meat of 70 degrees for at least ten minutes.

CUT OUT THE MOLD OR THROW IT AWAY

Particularly critical are aflatoxins, the most dangerous mold toxins for humans. They are considered cancerogenic. They are found mainly on and in vegetable, which contains a lot of fat or carbohydrates, for example in nuts. Aflatoxins are tasteless and not always recognizable.

At most a mold can give hints. The baking heat only partially destroys aflatoxins. As the fats of ground nuts are especially easy to rancid, you should not swallow them for atypical taste for safety's sake. Mold coverings can also be critical for other foods:

- Meat. Meat and sausage with mold always belongs completely in the bin.
- Dairy products. Also yogurt and quark should be disposed of immediately, if mold has formed.
- Jam. Throw away jam or marmalade if it has a mold. Only with a sugar content of more than 63 percent is it sufficient to lift off the mold stains generously.
- Loaf. Small, newly formed spots on bread loaves can cut out generously. Otherwise, throw it away better.
- Cheese. On or in blue cheese such as Camembert, Brie or Gorgonzola mold is of course desirable. If he transfers to sliced cheese, the rule is: throw away.
- Fruit and vegetables. For apples, it is enough to simply cut away fouling. Juicy ones like pears, peaches and tomatoes should be thrown away if they have formed fouling.

Tips For Shopping

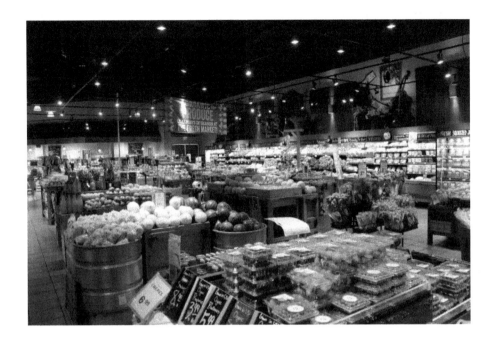

When shopping applies: Well-planned is usually already won. Anyone who thinks before, what he wants to cook buys more targeted and provides more variety.

Generally good: Buy fresh and seasonal goods as much as possible. It tastes better and is often cheaper.

FRUIT AND VEGETABLES

Season: Buy seasonally. Tomatoes, radishes or strawberries have a long journey in the winter and come mostly from the greenhouse. This is at the expense of taste and vitamin content.

Fresh or frozen: Let withered spinach or yellowish broccoli lie down. When in doubt, frozen vegetables are

better. It is processed harvest fresh, the vitamin content is higher and the taste better than long-stored goods. Sometimes the handle to preserve is worthwhile. Example tomatoes: Here come fully ripe fruit in the can.
Mature or immature: Ripe fruits give on finger pressure usually slightly and smell good. Some fruits and vegetables can also be bought immature. Apples, bananas, kiwis or avocados ripen at home.
Appearance: The appearance is often secondary: the shinier the apple, the more likely it has been treated with pesticides. You should also ignore size and commercial classes: Especially small fruits are often big in taste.
Packaged fruit: Should you weigh. For cardboard trays, check that the soil is moist. Then down is slush.
Street stalls. Small greengrocers often offer particularly appetizing greens. But you should intensively brush it at home. Car exhaust and abraded brake pads are deposited.

FISH

Storage: If possible, fresh fish should be on ice and covered with it. Also packaged smoked fish must be sufficiently cooled. As a precaution, do not buy goods that have almost reached the end of their shelf life.

Appearance and smell: Moist, bright red gills, shiny skin, clear mucus and clear eyes characterize fresh fish. If the fish smells severe, do without it.

Fish sticks: Are a viable alternative for anyone who likes neither the sight nor the taste of raw fish. They contain all essential ingredients. But: A stick is 35 percent breadcrumbs, which fat and energy levels grow enormously. Who wants to reduce the fat content, can bake the fish fingers in the oven.

Shellfish: Filtering with food also pollutants from the water. If possible, avoid mussels from near-industrial regions. Mussel meat spoils even easier than fish. Open mussels have to close on pressure themselves. Otherwise they should be sorted out.

Surimi: Is not an exquisite delicacy, but a crustacean or crabmeat from fish leftovers. It can also contain dyes and is flavored with sugar, salt and spices. Allergy sufferers should carefully examine the list of ingredients.

Sustainable fishing: The oceans are overfished. About half of the food fish comes from farms today (aquaculture). If you have wild fish, pay attention to the MSC seal or else opt for organic aquaculture.

MEAT

Appearance: Good meat should not be absolutely lean. A light marbling not only serves better cooking, but also the taste. Fresh meat should not be too light, too shiny, dry or too moist.

Self-service: Take a good look at meat: the blood on the bone must be fresh and bright red.

Cool. Meat spoils quickly at room temperature. That means go home quickly and put it in the refrigerator or prepare it.

Whitewashing: Sometimes the rosy fresh offer from the meat counter on the way home gets a pale, unappealing color. This may be due to the lighting in the counter. Anyone who believes that they have been "duped" should change the butcher.

CHEESE

Arrangement: Cheese should be arranged by kinship, i.e. hard and white and white mold with white cheese. Molds can migrate, and taste notes can influence them.

Aroma: Buy cheese in one piece. Pre-cut, it dries out and quickly loses its aroma. Press soft cheese lightly. Young cheese is firm, more mature gives way

Errors And Myths

They persist - find themselves regularly in the media or in conversations with friends and acquaintances:

supposedly clever truths. But few are proven. test.de puts some stubborn myths to the test.

"FRESH VEGETABLES HAVE MORE VITAMINS THAN THE ONES FROM THE FREEZER"

Partially correct: only true if the vegetables come straight out of the garden. In the supermarket shelf, fresh vegetables are often already a few days old and have already lost vitamins: for example, spinach can have up to 50 percent less vitamin C. Frozen spinach, on the other hand, contains about 30 percent less vitamin C than field-fresh spinach, but on average just as many B vitamins.

Frozen vegetables cannot beat just harvested vegetables, but in winter, when fresh food is scarce, it's a good choice. Tip: When thawing, you will save the light-, oxygen- and heat-sensitive vitamins if you cook the vegetables while still frozen and do not cook too long.

"FAT MAKES YOU FAT"

Right: With more than 9 kilocalories per gram, fat delivers significantly more energy than carbohydrates or protein, each with only 4 kilocalories per gram. In addition, the body can convert dietary fat to depot fat virtually one to one. By contrast, when converting carbohydrates or protein into body fat, around a quarter of the energy is lost.

Not correct: Fat does not saturate. The saturation effect may be delayed. However, studies have shown that the fat - once it's in the intestine and while it's there - inhibits the appetite for extra fat.

Also, many people stay slim and lean, even though they eat significantly more fat than diet societies recommend. You just save on other nutrients, such as carbohydrates from calories sweets.

Tip: Anything that you overeat - whether fat or sweet - beats down on your hips.

"BREAD IS A FAD"

Not correct: At least when it comes to whole meal bread. That contains a lot of fiber. And fiber contains virtually no calories. But they fill the intestines and make him a lot of work.

They have long-term satiety, are helpful in calorie saving. Also important: they regulate the bowel movement. The insoluble cellulose, for example, is practically not degraded by the intestinal bacteria and contributes to the brisk transport of the chyme. Hemicellulose and other soluble fibers swell up in the stomach and intestines, increase stool volume and stimulate intestinal activity. Additional plus: fiber promotes a healthy intestinal flora and some lower the cholesterol content in the blood. Although they are also in fruits and vegetables, but wholegrain bread is just a hit here.

Tip: When buying bread, make sure that you choose whole grains. In addition the cereals-product information under fruits and vegetables

"A LOT OF SALT LEADS TO HIGH BLOOD PRESSURE"

Partly correct: high blood pressure can be caused by increased salt consumption. That is not the only cause. And not every person reacts equally sensitively to salt. An estimated 40 percent of hypertensive patients are sensitive to salt - they lower their blood pressure when they consume less salt and vice versa.

This individual saline sensitivity probably has genetic causes. Since healthy people can also react sensitively to salt, the general rule is that there should not be more than six grams of table salt per day.

This is equivalent to a heaped teaspoon. Above all, junk food is often rich in salt.

Tip: With home-cooked you can determine the amount of salt yourself.

"COFFEE IS UNHEALTHY"

Wrong: For example, refutes now that coffee withdraws liquid. He acts only diuretic: Man excretes caffeinated drinks faster than caffeine-free, but not more than he drinks it. Cappuccino, espresso or milk coffee can therefore be included in the daily fluid balance.

Too much caffeine can make you nervous and restless. Even tremors and sleep disturbances can occur with too much coffee. It should therefore not be more than four cups of filter coffee a day.

Tip: Do not use dehydrating medication for weight loss. During a diet, drink extra - at least two liters per day.

"LATE FOOD MAKES YOU FAT"

Correct: Late evening gluttony leads to stomach pressure and affects the night's sleep.

Wrong: However, this does not make you necessarily thicker. On the one hand - unlike previously thought - the digestive system is also active at night. It may even be more active than during the day.

On the other hand, it has no influence on the calorie account when it is eaten. Example: Many slender Mediterranean settlers do not get up until the evening, eat until late at night - and eat rather sparsely.

Tip: It only counts how much you eat a day. Accordingly, you should calculate the calories.

"FIVE MEALS ARE IDEAL"

Partly correct: The saying is true for people whose blood sugar levels are always falling sharply. Several meals a day keep the sugar level in balance and constantly provide the brain with energy in the form of sugar. It does not tire so quickly. Food cravings stay out.

Obese people, on the other hand, are often better served with only three meals. Above all, they often have a disturbed sense of satiety. Overweight people tend to get too strong even with a snack. Your daily calorie account then has an undesirable plus.

Tip: Listen to your "belly" and decide for yourself how many meals are needed for your figure and your well-being.

"COLA AND PRETZEL STICKS HELP WITH DIARRHEA"

Wrong: This home remedy is by no means optimal. In diarrhea, the body loses water and electrolytes, so salts such as potassium. To balance the loss of fluids and minerals, the body needs the right mix of salts and sugar.

Cola consists of eleven percent sugar; this amount increases the loss of water. Potassium is barely contained, and the caffeine in the cola encourages the kidneys to further potassium excretion. Pretzel sticks are ok, but they are mostly sodium and not potassium.

Tip: In case of diarrhea are more suitable electrolyte mixtures from the pharmacy or with salt and sugar enriched juice spritzers, to stomach-friendly food such as rusk or crushed banana

Chapter 9   Muscle Growth Requirements

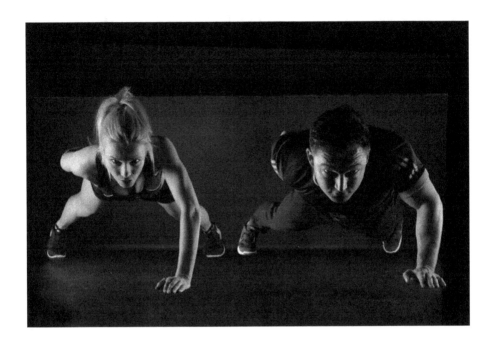

Muscle growth requirements are essentially what's required in your training to build an adequate amount muscle within a set time span. For the average person with a male or female one can build anywhere between one anywhere between 20 to 30 pounds of muscle within the first year depending on your gender, nutrition, sleep, workout routine and effectiveness. The process gets slower over time so essentially you will be putting on a one to two pounds after 4-5 years. And then after that each a more advanced stage know probably half a pound a year.

So, it's a process you need to know once you follow requirements like sleep requirements are on point and you are working hard in gym and you're consistent with your workouts and in the gym or working out anywhere between two to three times a week on every body part with adequate rest is then you're definitely on track to building 40- 50 pounds of lean muscle within a five-year period which is a great accomplishment for anybody.

A strong and disciplined mind is necessary to see optimal results. This is not an overnight process and requires patience on your part. Many beginners will give up 3 months or less when they don't see proper or any noticeable results either stemming from too high body fat, terrible nutrition, sleep, smoking, alcohol, stress you name it. Time can be both friend and enemy depending on you use it. So, stay patient follow the necessary guidelines and results will come flying your way.

When first starting out you can expect neural fatigue or extreme tiredness will be a normal thing. This response is a result of your body trying to adapt to the hard work and stress on muscles and nervous system. It just means your immune system is working overtime because it's very weak because you your body has to throw all your energy our resources into lifting heavier weight and doing more hectic things. Over time your body will adapt to doing this over the course of 3-5 months and working out will be the norm for your body. So, don't be deterred by small problems that might occur learn to adapt to your environs

Bear all those things in mind prior to getting into bodybuilding it's something that will have to become a lifestyle to see maximum gains.

CARDIO

Cardio is a mixture of cardio and body weight training. Most of your muscle building should focused on your body weight and weight training as too much cardio can be detrimental to your muscle gain as it may cause you to lose muscle and in that case I would recommend anywhere between two to three times a week for cardio preferably if it can be done after your exercises or days you won't be working out so it doesn't hamper your ability to work out.

Cardio is still beneficial to your training as it keeps your body in a state where you're able to last longer essentially in the gym right because your heart is strong and it's able to pump blood more efficient and so leading to higher endurance one exercises.

Added benefits of cardio include:

1.   Improves cardiovascular health

2.   Improves mood [can have an effect on your strength training especially]

3.   Helps regulate blood sugar

4.   Reduces chronic pain

5.   Aids sleep [Beneficial for workouts]

6.   Regulates weight [aid in building leaner muscles]

7.   Improves brain power [Which translates to good workout performance

Cardio has its place in the gym if used properly with weight, body-weight and strength training.

BODYWEIGHT TRAINING

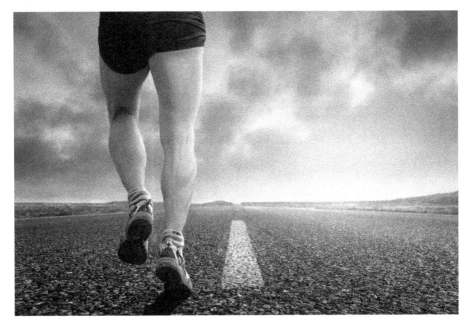

Body weight and weightlifting in general are the main exercises to build serious muscle. Body weight exercises as the name suggests are a group of exercises that require you to use you lift your body weight. These movements influence hypertrophy and can improve fitness and flexibility if done right.

The most popular body weight exercises would be push-ups and pull-ups which tend to be the more standard of the two also dips are a good one. Dips and pull-ups do tend to be more intermediate in the sense that you're not able to do them of the bat when starting out as a beginner especially if you have no experience with them. So, it's generally best to start off with push-ups preferably if you can do anywhere between 10 to 20 push-ups about 5 sets. When the exercise gets easier using a weight on your back can assist also having a very light person either exert pressure or actually sit on your back.

In terms of hardness push-ups are relatively easy even for a beginner who generally should be able to do at least 3-5 at a normal weight. If you're overweight this might prove a challenge for you. So, doing them on your knees is a good way to start out until you can do them fully up on your feet.

Body weight training is recommended for beginners especially who want an idea of what lifting weight feels like prior to going into the harder stuff like weight and strength training.

Push-ups [Chest exercise]

Pull-ups [Back exercise]

Dips [Triceps]

Dips [Chest]

WEIGHT TRAINING

Weight training this is where things get a bit more complicated. For beginners I recommend buying a gym membership and finding a good gym. This ensures you can learn to do the exercises properly from professionals in your vicinity. Make an effort to go to the gym at least four to five days a week as a beginner you want to have maximal frequency as far as going to the gym is concerned as this is where you make most of your gains and you want your body to adjust to the strain that you'll be putting it under.

The frequency of your gym time can be dropped down over the span of a year or two to maybe three times or even two times a week. In my case I prefer doing two full body exercises for the week and then the days in between that I'll do a mixture of upper body and lower body exercises to fill the gap. As a beginner I recommend doing split meaning one day work certain parts of your body or your whole upper body another day working your lower body. So, a good example of workout days is Monday are my arms [biceps and my triceps]. I'm going to discuss some exercises for those later on so biceps and triceps and I'm also going to be doing my chest and back and shoulders that is like bench presses and rows and so forth. Then Wednesday I work my legs [quadriceps, hamstrings and calves and butt]. Friday upper body again. Then Saturday lower body like Wednesday and start this over the following week with at least one to two rest days in between. And let's not forget your good ole forearms which can be worked using reverse bicep curls, hammer curls,

As far as exercises go, we're going to start with the upper body and specifically the arms. Great bicep exercises are seated or standing bicep curls or hammer curls and preacher curls. All those exercises are great for isolating the biceps. A good workout set is 4 sets of 12 on any of these or perhaps doing "21s" where you basically do 7 full reps, 7 half reps down and 7 half reps up. For triceps you have tricep pulldowns, close grip bench press, tricep kickbacks, skull crushers and the list goes on. As with biceps these exercises are great for isolating the triceps which are made up of 3 heads which get hit based on how each is done something. The last arm muscle would be the forearms a muscle which is typically ignored by many beginners. The forearms consist of 4 different muscles each with a job to either turn the arm, grip objects or lift the arm. Great exercises for the forearms include wrist rotators, reverse curl [instead of underhand grip overhand], farmer's walk, wrist rotations etcetera. The forearms can be worked with the same frequency and rep ranges as the biceps. In order to have a truly massive arm forearms can't be neglected especially if you have smaller wrists, they give a great big hand illusion and since your forearms show more than your upper arm, they will be the main one seen so work those bad boys! Next, we have shoulders and as with the triceps the shoulder consists of three heads the front deltoids, side deltoids and rear deltoids. Each head is worked based on the variety of shoulder exercise. But a key thing to note is any push movement in front like the bench press or even overhead press will hit the front head, the side head which arguable is the weakest head can be hit using any side or lateral raising movements and the back head which is a bit trickier to work is worked by any pulling movements like face pulls, dumbbell raises done with your upper body facing forward and your face to the ground and so forth.

Next, we have the chest and some common chest exercises include, barbell bench press, dumbbell bench press, cable flies, seated flies, pushups or weighted pushups and most pushing movements that push your arms out in front of you will target the chest.

Next, we have the back which is made up of several muscles. From top to bottom we have the trapezius muscles [muscles on both sides of your neck], which can be worked using shrugs behind or in front the body with barbells and even dumbbell shrugs, deadlift to a degree hits them. Then you have your minor rhomboid and major rhomboid which make up your center back, these can be worked using, most pull movements like barbell or dumbbell rows, pullbacks or even T-bar rows are great for building thickness. Then we have the Latissimus dorsi or the "lats" as they're famously called which give your back that wideness and add to your V-taper. These can be worked mainly using pull-ups, cable pull downs etcetera. Then you have your lower back which is a part of your core and aids in stability of the entire body these can be worked using deadlifts, more lighter exercises include bridges, knee to chest and lateral leg lifts and plank holds. Deadlift hands down are one of the best back exercises since they target several back muscles including other muscles like your legs and arms.

Next, we move onto lower body. From top to bottom we have the glutes or the buttocks, quadriceps, hamstrings and calves. A nice workout set for these could be first starting with the bigger muscle groups. So, a variety of butt, and upper leg exercises. First, we'll start with hamstring which is in my opinion the most attractive leg muscle as it can be seen from the front. Exercises for the quads include; squats [barbell front and back], Bulgarian split squats, goblet squat etcetera. For the hamstrings you have; deadlifts [believe it or not this a full body and it destroys the hamstrings just as much as the back- in a good way of course], leg curls [with a machine], glute-ham raise, walking lunges, etcetera. For the glutes you have; band hip thrusters, band kickbacks, deadlifts [of course you'd be here], squats [can't forget good ole squats], kettlebell swings etcetera. And last but not least, good ole calves. As with forearms and rear deltoids these tend to be neglected by a lot of beginners even some advanced bodybuilders. Good calf exercises include; double or single leg raise preferably standing with the sole of your feet hanging off a step or a something you can stand on and hold on to something else whilst raising your legs into a tip toe position stretching your calves at the top and bottom, box jumps, seated calf raises, tip toe walk [don't drop your heels on the floor whilst walking] etcetera.

A good workout sets for each of these leg muscles is 3-4 sets of 6-12 reps depending on your goals. If it's hypertrophy 8-12 is a good rep range [the calves can work with 16-20]. Another thing to bear in mind is squats are a good full-body exercises and as far as the lower body is concerned, glutes, hamstrings, quads and a little calves are hit hard when you do front or back squats. So, try your best to incorporate that beast into you all your leg routines and deadlift if you can also.

Strength Training

So, strength training is training which generally pushes the muscular and more importantly the neuro system more than normal in order to lift more weight. Your muscles and also your entire body play a huge role in providing resources to lift. In strength training your muscles essentially recoup more resources from the body than normally need to achieve the desired goal. There are certain exercises which are generally considered more strength related exercises so for example your 4 main compound exercises like your bench-press, squat, overhead press or OVP and your deadlift will tend to be usual suspects for strength training. Those exercises will generally push your body beyond what it's comfortable with as you progressively overload the weight. Your typical isolation exercises can also be strength based like your dumbbell curls and dumbbell press but they don't give your overall physic the type of strength more compound or full body movements can since these require more muscles to push the weight and can be done with more weight.

A key recommendation with strength training is to progressively overload your muscles. This means try and add 5-10 pounds on the bar based on which ever exercise you're doing. The strongest lift should be your deadlift and strength gains for natural bodybuilders slow down around 500+ so maybe 5- 10 pounds every month or couple months depending on your overall weightlifting requirements met [so calories intake, type of calories, supplementation, sleep etcetera].

An important caveat to note with strength training is unless you're training for a strongman type competition the risk to reward is probably not worth it because as you go over certain weight amounts like for example over 315 on bench depending on your build can start to stress your joints over time especially as a natural bodybuilder who isn't taking drugs specifically meant to aid in joint density and protection. That being said progressively overloading or lifting heavier as you get stronger is not inherently bad as this allows you to overcome some plateaus you may face as certain weights become too easy for you to handle. The problem comes into play when your main focus is getting very strong with no real goal but to look strong in the gym; but to each his own, I guess.

My recommendation is if strength isn't your main goal and you're not competition prepping mixing a bit of strength training with your normal weight training routine can help you to make some great gains in both departments. So, for example some if you work out 4 days a week allocate 2 days where you do heavy and the other two a mix of light to medium. So, a good regimen is Monday heavy bench and squat, Wednesday light to medium lower body, Friday heavy overhead press and deadlift and then Saturday is a medium to light upper body day. So, it's about mixing and matching and working out smart. I generally avoid mixing deadlift and squats on the same day since they both tax the lower back. The same also applies with bench and overhead press they both tax the anterior chain of the shoulders or the front deltoids so doing them on different days helps.

Chapter 10   The Glycemic Index and Bodybuilding Nutrition

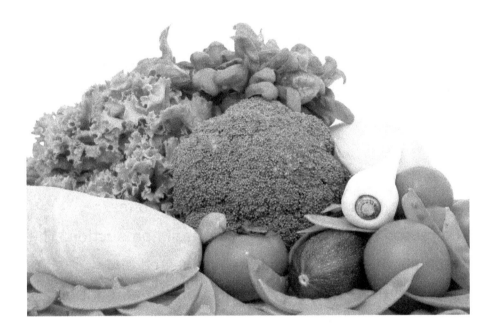

We often hear about the GI, or glycemic index. It measures the rate at which your blood glucose level rises after you eat a carbohydrate. Put simply, when you eat a carbohydrate of some description, it is digested and converted to glucose or blood sugar. The body uses the glucose to make ATP – Adenosine Tri-Phosphate – which is needed to power the functions of the body and act as the fuel it needs to function properly.

Each carbohydrate is given a GI value ranging from zero to 100. That value is based on how quickly your blood glucose levels rise within two hours after eating the food. A food that has a value of one raises the glucose level very quickly, whereas a low number indicates a food that takes longer to raise the glucose level. Mid-range numbers take a moderate amount of time. When it comes to controlling fat loss and the rate at which your blood sugar rises, it is best to go for the mid-range foods instead of the high-end ones.

The reason for this goes down to insulin production. The speed at which a carbohydrate is digested and converted to glucose has an effect on the amount of insulin released to control the glucose levels. If the food converts to glucose too quickly, your insulin levels will go through the roof, which is not a good situation for a person who is looking to lose body fat. High insulin levels are not conducive to fat loss; instead, they simply force the fat into storage. A food that releases the glucose slowly will result in less insulin and a higher chance of burning off fat.

So when it comes to bodybuilding and fat loss, is the glycemic index important? Yes and no. It is important to understand the effect that different foods have on your glucose levels. A number of studies have been conducted, and they reached the conclusion that consuming carbohydrates with a low GI throughout the course of a day will suppress the appetite and keep energy levels steady.

Moreover, low GI foods allow you to eat more without storing body fat and supporting fat loss. However, GI is not the only thing that affects body fat storage.

What Are Low GI Foods?

There are lots of different thoughts on what a low GI food is – anything with a score of less than 55 is generally thought to be low, between 55 and 70 is medium, and above that is considered high. However, you have to take into account the foods that you consume with those carbohydrates because they, too, will have an effect on your GI. Whenever you eat proteins with carbohydrates, the GI value of the meal drops because protein is considered a complex molecule that slows down the rate at which the carbohydrate is digested. Fats also do the same thing. Thus, given that there is little chance that you will only be eating carbohydrates, the G number is only to be used as a guide. Also, the glycemic index doesn't tell us the whole story; it doesn't tell us the best carbs to eat if we want to lose fat.

One of the biggest reasons why we can't use the glycemic index as the sole measure of choosing the right carbohydrates is that GI does not account for how the human body handles simple carbohydrates against complex carbohydrates.

Complex And Simple Carbohydrates

All carbohydrates fall into one of two categories – simple or complex. The complex carbohydrate is made up of numerous units of sugar, all linked up in single molecules. This is why they are called "complex." They tend to provide a level of energy that is sustained as long as their GI value is low to medium. A high GI value complex carbohydrate will act like a simple carbohydrate being digested very quickly.

There are two different types of complex carbohydrate, each of which you should be eating in small portions at frequent intervals throughout the day:

- Starchy – these provide raw energy that the body can make good use of. Excellent sources of these are brown rice, grits, lentils, oatmeal, cream of wheat, and sweet potatoes

- Fibrous – these cannot be absorbed by the body but are packed full of minerals and vitamins. On top of that, the fiber is excellent for helping to clean the intestines, thus allowing the nutrients you get from the more digestible foods to be absorbed better. If you mix a starchy complex carb with a fibrous one, it will decrease the speed at which the starchy carb is digested, once again lowering the GI value of that food. Excellent sources are cherries, asparagus pears, apples, oranges, cantaloupes, grapefruit, strawberries, nectarines, lemons, and peaches. After a workout, try to eat the high-sugar foods, such as bananas or grapes.

The Simple Carbohydrate And The Effect It Has On Body Fat

Most fruits have a low GI number, but fruits contain a simple sugar called fructose, which is metabolized in a way completely different from that of the sugars found in starchy foods. To understand the process, you first need to understand the way the body uses glucose. When your blood sugar levels are low, the body will make use of any glucose it gets from the food you consume, and it will burn it straightaway for fuel. This is why, when you have finished a workout, your body will make very efficient use of carbohydrates. Now, let's assume that you do not have a real need for energy. In that scenario, the glucose you consume would then be converted into glycogen, which gets stored in your muscles or liver. Your liver is able to hold about 100 grams of glycogen, but your muscle can hold between 200 and 400 grams, depending, of course, on how muscular you are.

There is a key point here that you must remember – glycogen that is stored in your muscles can only supply the muscles with energy when they are contracting, which is why your muscle glycogen stores tend to be badly depleted while you are working out. The glycogen in your liver, on the other hand, can supply your whole body with energy, and this is what you have to remember in order to grasp why fructose doesn't help you burn off fat.

When you eat an excessive amount of carbohydrates, your body will only get fat if all of your glycogen stores are full up. The extra glucose that cannot be stored will be converted into fat by the liver and then gets stored as body fat, or adipose tissue, usually in the buttocks, thighs, and abdomen. When you eat foods that are high in fructose, the muscles are lacking the enzyme that is required to convert the fructose into glycogen. The liver, however, does have this enzyme, and that means the fructose serves to replenish your liver. However, it doesn't take that much to replenish the liver because, as I said earlier, it only holds around 100 g of glycogen. This means that if you eat too much fruit, your liver stores will fill up quickly, and this will force the body to produce phosphofructokinase. This is an enzyme that tells the body that all the glycogen stores are full and can take no more. Given that the liver is responsible for supplying the whole body with energy, the glycogen stores are seen as a fuel gauge. When the tank is full up, extra fuel is stored elsewhere and, because of this, it is suggested that you keep your fruit intake to a minimum, even eliminating them from your diet altogether if your diet is one that is aiming for aggressive fat loss. For those of you that are wondering how a low GI food, such as fruit, can do so much damage, it's because when the fructose leaves the liver, it does so as fat, and that will not raise your insulin levels.

Recommendations for the Consumption of Carbohydrates

For a proper nutritional bodybuilding diet, we recommend that you stick to carbohydrates that have a GI value of 64 or less throughout the day. These will create a consistent level of energy to aid in daily function and peak performance. If you do have to eat fruit, keep your servings down to no more than two a day, and eat them when the liver is depleted of glycogen – first thing in the morning and straight after a workout are the best times.

How to Benefit from Old-School Habits

We often hear that we are exactly what we eat and, to be honest, this is very true. You can look at just about anybody and determine if they eat a healthy nutritious diet or one that is full of processed high-sugar junk. Obesity is one of the biggest growing problems (pardon the pun), and it is starting to affect our children. There are dozens of TV reality shows about people who are looking to drop the pounds, programs on obesity, and those that cover the medical effects, such as diabetes. If you are old enough, take a look back to the 1970s. Do you remember if obesity was that much of a problem then? Did we see all these shows? Were there all these diseases around? The answer is no. I'm not, for one minute, suggesting that it didn't happen; I'm just saying that we never saw it so much. These days, we live a life on the run, grabbing a bite to eat here and there. Most of these foods are convenience or junk, and we never stop to think about the bad fat or sugar content or the effect it will have on us – at least, not until the scale has jumped by 100 lbs or more.

In the 70s, schools took a bit more pride in what they served kids in the cafeteria. The meals were properly balanced and tasted good. Today's meals are bland, packaged meals that are next to useless.

Back then, a bodybuilder diet consisted of a lot of protein and a little carbohydrate. The protein was used to help build up the muscle, and the lower level of carbs was designed to reduce the amount of body fat. This diet was coupled with supplements, such as liver pills, which would build up the gases in the stomach, and soy protein (which, in all honesty, wasn't that good).

Protein powders made their debut in stores, and many bodybuilders used to take extra protein in the form of dehydrated fish power. It didn't get digested very easily, and it tasted foul, but it did have some value.

The diet was pretty much a "real food" diet, that is, a basic one like this:

Breakfast – three eggs, a beef patty, cottage cheese, and some vitamins

Lunch – fish, chicken, or another beef patty, a small salad, with optional eggs, cottage cheese, or tuna

Snack – chicken breast, a can of tuna, or a protein drink

Dinner – chicken or steak, small salad, cottage cheese, vegetables, and sugar-free jello

Bedtime snack – a cheese omelet

This was a high-protein, low-carb diet with the fat coming from cream, extra rich milk, or eggs. These fats were used as a fuel by bodybuilders in training because they would not be stored in the body, whereas the carbohydrates are stored and then burned off later on. A certain amount of calories had to be burned off, and fat intake would increase this number. However, going too long with limited carbohydrate intake only depletes the brain and body, and it can have a detrimental effect on your mood and induce anger as well.

You need a certain amount of sugar and, for one day a week, the diet would be pushed to one side. This was the "cheat day" – a day when anything could be eaten, regardless of how "junky" it was. The belief back then was that you could eat as much as you wanted because it wasn't possible to get fat in just one day. All you ate would never stick, passing right through you, only retaining water, and pushing your weight up by a few pounds. Water weight is the first to shift so, within a couple of days, your weight would go back down again. Today, we are told that we must be careful how much fat we eat because it can raise cholesterol levels and cause heart disease. To be fair, too much of a good thing is not always a good thing but is perfectly okay in moderation. Later on in the 70s, the Atkins diet appeared, along with a few other fad diets that were nothing more than copies of the bodybuilder diet of the day. The biggest issues with this kind of diet were the swings in mood and the feeling of being starved of carbohydrates. Elimination was an issue because of the low level of fiber and high level of protein. A little bit of sugar would balance the mood, and a small helping of fiber a couple of times a day would sort out the other issues.

Using a diet like this can have you looking lean and feeling fit in no time at all. Stop the diet and go back, and you might be shocked at how quick the weight goes back on, which, in some cases, would be more than you lost in the first place. In terms of bodybuilding, this diet – the diet of the 70s – is fine if you use it in moderation. Ditch the cheat day, so you are not eating high-carb foods nonstop for several hours. Instead, eat a few more carbs every day. Space your meals out evenly, and if you feel like you are putting on a pound or two, scale back on the carbs a little.

At the end of the day, for a successful bodybuilding program and a great physique, eat a healthy balanced diet, drink plenty of water, and keep on training. Remember that good fat is your friend, and fruit may well be considered your enemy!

Chapter 11   Bodybuilding Nutrition the Simple Way

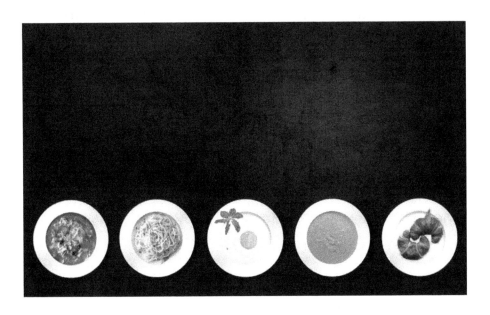

Most bodybuilders are aware that they have to eat a diet that is full of the right nutrition if they want the best body, but they are not always entirely sure where to begin. Nutrients appear to be somewhat mysterious and a little complex but, in all honesty, they are not. Provided you start from the top and work downwards, nutrients are very simple to understand.

Much of the confusion seems to come from people who say that you "must do it this way" or "you should be eating this and not that." Much of what you hear ends up causing confusion, and nothing seems to fit, making it very difficult to see the big picture. This is why I am going to show you the big picture and let you sort out your own nutrition to meet the goals that you have set. Think of your nutritional plan as being something like a personal household budget. Both plans are all about making the right choice, even if it is a difficult one, and then sticking to it. Blow the budget, and disaster is waiting. The same goes for your nutrition plan – deviate from it, and everything you have done will be lost. When you draw up a financial plan, you begin with your income. You subtract any expenses that have to be paid to work out what your spending amount is. When you draw up a nutritional plan, you begin with the number of calories you can consume in a day, subtracting everything that is needed for lean muscle growth. This will tell you the amount of cheat foods you can have.

How To Draw Up A Nutritional Bodybuilding Plan

Step 1 – Work out your calorie requirements per day

This is your starting point, and it will take you no more than a couple of minutes to work out. Use a calorie counter to work out the energy requirements of your body on a daily basis. This is your TDEE, or Total Daily Energy Expenditure. For example, a 25-year-old who weighs 160 lb, stands 68 inches tall, and works out for three to five hours a week doing cardio will have a TDEE of 2721 calories on a daily basis.

Step 2 – Determine your caloric goal

What is your goal here? Is it bulking up, cutting out, or recompositioning? If you are cutting, your caloric goal per day will be lower than your TDEE. If you are bulking up, it will be higher than your TDEE, while recompositioning means that your caloric goal must match your TDEE exactly. Let's go back to the person in step 1. He wants to cut so his caloric goal will be a deficit of 20%; 2721 calories less 20% is equal to 2176 calories per day.

Step 3 – Determine your Macro

Macro is a shortened version of Macronutrient Ratios. In the bodybuilding world, this can be one of these nutritional pigeonholes – fat, carbohydrate, and protein. What you need to determine would be the percentages of calories that you will allocate to each of these three. Be aware that we calculate these percentages by calories, not by weight. Protein and carbohydrates are each 4 calories a gram, while fat is 9 calories. Some of the more common macros are:

40/40/20 – 40% protein, 40% carbohydrate, 20% fat

40/50/10 – 40% protein, 50% carbohydrate, 10% fat

50/10/40 – 50% protein, 10% carbohydrate, 40% fat

It isn't always a good idea to set your protein on a percentage level though; it is much better if you base it on your body weight. As a rule, it is recommended that you consume 1 gram of protein for each pound of body weight. A 200 lb person would eat 200 grams of protein. So, what would that be in terms of percentages? Well, that depends on how much cardio exercise you do. If you do none at all, you might have to go up as high as 40% protein to make sure you get that 1 gram per pound. On the other hand, if you do loads of cardio, you could drop to as low as 20%. It isn't as complicated as it sounds if you use the right calorie calculator. Failing that, you can sit and work it out for yourself – once you've done it a few times, it'll become second nature to you.

Step 4 – Work out your budget

Now, with those macro percentages, you can work out your carbohydrate, protein, and fat intake in grams per day. Let's say that your caloric goals are 2176 per day. You set your ratios at 30/40/30. That means you would need to eat 653 calories of protein, 870 calories of carbohydrates, and 653 calories of fat per day. To work this out, you need to do a little bit of math. Fat contains 9 calories per gram, while protein and carbohydrates are both 4 calories per gram. To work out your grams:

653 calories of protein – 653/4 = 163 grams

870 calories of carbohydrates – 870/4 – 217 grams

653 calories of fat – 653/9 = 72 grams

These are your daily allowances for protein carbohydrate, and fat, and have to stick to these. With these figures, you can work out what foods you can and can't eat.

Is that it?

Sadly not. What would happen if you decided that you were going to stick to your macros but eat a large spoon of white refined sugar as your carbohydrate, a large bowl of isolated soy as your protein, and a big lump of margarine for your fat? This is just an example, and it is clearly not a very healthy one. There are other things that are just as important as fat, carbs, and protein when you are bodybuilding.

Antioxidants and Vitamins

Vitamins are vital for muscle building and, while you can get them in pill form, you are better off getting them from your food, which is a more natural and far better source. There are those who take a multivitamin everyday as a way of kidding themselves that they don't need to eat properly, and that is a particularly bad idea. Vegetables are the best form of vitamins, and they also contain fiber. Fiber is filling, and it contains no calories so you can cut your weight without ever having to feel hungry and deprived. Every day, eat between four and six cups of vegetables and three pieces of fruit. Go for the color – red or black grapes, berries, kale, red bell peppers, spinach, etc., to make sure you are getting the full dose of antioxidants as well.

- Fiber

As I mentioned earlier, fiber is an important part of any diet because it can help burn that fat off. Fiber contains absolutely no calories, but it is one of the most filling components of any diet, which means the more you eat, the less hungry you feel. This has the effect of lowering your calorie consumption. Fruits and vegetables are the main bearers of fiber, but eating those alone is simply not enough. You need to add beans and whole grains to your diet to make it up to 40 grams per day.

Omega-3 Fatty Acid

We all know that essential fatty acids are good for us, and the reason they are essential is because the human body cannot make them. There are two main essential fatty acids – linoleic acid or omega-6 and alpha-linoleic (ALA), which is omega-3. Omega-3 is more important, and you can find it in oily fish, such as salmon, mackerel, herring, and anchovies, as well as in flax seed. Omega-3 fatty acids are good for helping to protect the heart from disease and for improving brain function and preventing depression. In terms of bodybuilding, omega-3 fatty acids help you to gain the muscle mass you are seeking. The recommended dose is 5 mg per day, but you should try to get it from real food sources. If you have to take it in supplement form, go for a high-quality fish oil supplement.

High Quality Protein

I know I already mentioned this earlier, but I want to stress the importance of the quality of the protein you include in your diet. The most important part here is to balance out your protein needs across the food groups and your macros. If, while you are eating your protein allowance, you blow out the other macros, then your food budget is shot to pieces. Let's say that you choose fried chicken as your main source of protein, or perhaps you went for the Big Mac. You would almost certainly destroy your allowance for saturated fat and blow your fat macro out of the water. You must stick with lean protein sources. Even if a meat looks lean, it can contain a high level of fat, so take that into account when planning your meals.

High-quality protein is the key to growing big muscles and to getting stronger. While plant proteins are not as high in quality as that from meat source, there are other combinations that work. Milk and eggs contain the same, if not higher, quality of protein than chicken does.

- Good Fats

For so long, we have been told by the medical professionals that fat is bad for us, in all its forms. It seems that now, they are coming around to a way of thinking that most of us have known for years – some fats are good for you. MUFA – monounsaturated fat – and PUFA – polyunsaturated fat – are good for you. In their oil form, these types of fat are liquid when at room temperature but, instead of going for liquid oils, look for other sources. Nuts, avocados, and olives are some of the best sources of unsaturated good fat, and you should aim to get at least 10% of your calories every day from these fats.

For many years, high cholesterol was linked to the cholesterol that you consumed, but this has now been pushed to one side because it simply isn't true.

Saturated fat used to a big villain but, although you should aim to keep it down to less than 5% of your calories, it isn't as bad as it was once thought. The best place to get your saturated fats from is eggs, but be careful how many you eat. If you are eating eggs as your protein source, you must remove the yolk, as that is where the fat is.

The bad fats – the ones you really must avoid at all costs – are the ones that are factory-produced and those with long, complicated, chemical-like names. If you saw an ingredient called "partially hydrogenated vegetable oil," it's bad for you. Virtually any fried food you get from a fast food joint is bad because they are fried in that type of fat, and virtually all snacks and junk food also contain these types of fat.

Cheat Meals

So, what's left? We've got all the good stuff, so what you can have for your cheat meals? There is some good news and some bad news here. The good news is for those who are bulking or who have a surplus of calories over their TDEE – you have quite a bit of room to have some of those cheat meals. A candy bar, a beer, cake, and cookies are all okay so long as they fit in with your daily budget. The bad news is for those who are cutting. You have very little room left for cheats once you have satisfied all of your daily nutritional needs. In the example above where the person is at a 20% deficit, your cheat meal would be something worthless like half of a candy bar.

The truth about cheat meals and snacks is that a bodybuilder can actually lose fat and make muscle gains by incorporating a cheat meal into his or her diet. This is because if you followed your bodybuilding diet perfectly all the time, your body would become used to the caloric intake and, as a result, lowers its metabolism (caloric burning ability) in an effort to maintain the status quo. There are a couple of ways you can avoid this.

Caloric Cycling: This method allows you to keep your healthy eating habits intact. Simply up the calorie intake over the weekend, mainly in the form of good carbohydrates, before and after your work out to spike your metabolism.

Once a Week Cheat Meal: Another way you can avoid the slowing of your metabolism is to introduce a cheat meal into your diet. If you constantly crave a specifically forbidden food, this may be a good way to satisfy those cravings while accomplishing the goal of increasing your metabolism. The keys to making a cheat meal work are to plan ahead on what you're going to eat and to employ portion control measures. For example, your cheat meal cannot be three gallons of ice cream topped with hot fudge. Also, limit the cheat meal to one hour, unless it is Thanksgiving or Christmas, in which case a cheat day is acceptable. Keep in mind that if you eat everything you can see without restraint, the chances are that any benefit you could have gained from the cheat meal will be lost, as it may take a whole week to burn off all the calories you have consumed. In this case, your fat loss results will also be compromised. Therefore, you must use common sense and self-control for you cheat meal to work.

Anyone with 20% body fat or higher should use extreme caution when meal cheating. If you fall into this category, the size and frequency of your cheat meal should be very minimal. This is because if you are overweight, there is a good chance that your metabolism is much slower than that of your thinner counterparts, which means that you have a greater probability of having most of those extra calories from your cheat meal converted into body fat.

So hopefully, you've got the idea and can now work out your own daily nutritional budget. For every single calorie that you need to eat, ask yourself how to get the most for it. Instead of eating the empty calories in a candy bar, go for an apple that contains vitamins and fiber, as well as a small handful of peanuts for the good fats. Nutrition is all about making the small decisions on what to eat and all of them add up.

Chapter 12   Bodybuilding Mistakes To Avoid

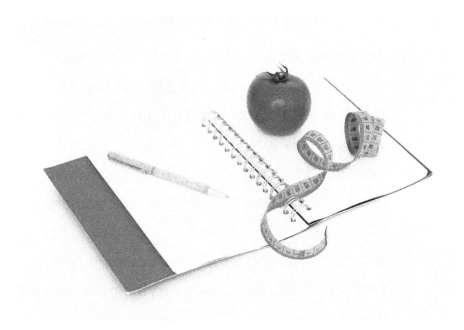

In addition to workout fatigue, bodybuilders should also be careful about other things and activities that can ruin their physique or health. The following are common mistakes of bodybuilders that you should avoid:

- Eating a lot. Excess calories will become fat. That means if you have consumed excessive calories, you also have to do excessive workouts. It may sound fun, but too much of a good thing is bad. Overtraining can lead to muscle fatigue and could affect your performance in the long run. Eating just the right amount of food with enough calories to burn is always recommended.

- Eating too little. You may think that since overeating is bad, you will just eat less to make sure that you don't get fat. However, eating less is just as bad as eating a lot. If your diet lacks essential nutrients, how can you build muscles? Remember that you are a bodybuilder, not a model of slimming supplements. You should always have enough protein, carbs, and fats. Everything works well with balance.

- Insufficient protein intake. Yes, you need three of them, protein, carbs, and fats. But the single most important nutrient for muscle building and rebuilding is protein. You might think it's easy since a lot of foods in the market have protein. The tricky part is that you have to eat lean protein, which is a little challenging to find.

- Not being able to cook for yourself. A successful bodybuilder knows how to prepare his food. Since you are fully conscious of what you eat, you should have time to learn what foods work best for your body. That means learning how to prepare them as well. Of course, this also comes with the willingness to do the actual meal preparations.

- Excessive fat and sugar. Both of these are the enemies of bodybuilders especially in excessive amounts. Fat has a lot of calories per gram compared to protein and carbs. It cannot be stressed enough that excess calories that are not burned turn into fat stores. The same is true with excess sugar. Always check the food labels for both low fat and low sugar products. Low fat milk with high sugar content will just be the same as milk with normal fat content.

- Insufficient water. It's the most basic of all lessons. You have to drink enough water to keep yourself hydrated. Even school kids are taught that the body is 67% water. Your teacher might also have told you to drink 8 glasses of water a day. Water keeps your body clean and flushes away unnecessary wastes and toxins.   When you do your workouts, you sweat as part of the body's self-cooling mechanism. Without sufficient water, your body will not be able to do this and you will feel the strain of your workouts sooner.

- Not taking supplements. Besides lifting weights, drinking water, and eating a proper diet, taking supplements is essential to becoming a good bodybuilder. Boosting your intake of muscle building nutrients will also boost the results of your workouts. Supplements help you gain that awesome physique faster. They help round out the nutrients you have absorbed from food. Even the greatest athletes have taken supplements one way or another. Serious bodybuilders take supplements which have higher loads of protein and carbs to aid in faster recovery time and therefore, more workout capacity.

Conclusion

Successful bodybuilders believe that your goals are reached in your mind first – mind over body. If you can see it, you can achieve it. There you have it – almost everything you need to know about bodybuilding to make an informed decision about whether this is what you want to do. It is a life-long lifestyle change that requires dedication and commitment. Make your decision, and stick to it. Have your goals mapped out, and gun for them.

Make small changes and build confidence in your ability to reach that goal. This important step in your life is about the journey, not the result. If you are cooking for or with family members, involve them in the meal planning, shopping, and cooking.

Hopefully all your meal prep questions are answered and you can feel confident moving forward! Let's just briefly touch on some key items shared about earlier. Remember meal prepping is that it should be fun! Search out ways to make your meal prepping experience enjoyable. Bond with your family and friends, create a meal prep calendar, and share recipes with other meal peppers!

Also, watch what you put in your recipes. You want meal prepping to help your household become less processed. When you are shopping for your ingredients, try to buy all natural and organic ingredients. At the very least, read the ingredients on every can and jar you buy. Even something as simple as diced tomatoes can contain harmful additives like high fructose corn syrup. This can greatly change the nutrition facts of your recipe without you even knowing! Learn to become a master at reading labels. Choose the product that has the least amount of ingredients added in.

One can find meal prepping, a convenient, and cost-effective way of preparing your food. Instead of waking up early every time to prepare breakfast as well as cook for dinnertime after a hard day's work, you can easily pull out your ready-made meals anytime and enjoy eating a healthy clean meal.

This will not only be convenient but will likewise teach you how to organize your meals without the hassles of planning and cooking every day. You can organize everything from purchasing your kitchen supplies, containers, storage facilities, and more than everything – your time which is a valuable commodity.

Most bodybuilders are aware that they have to eat a diet that is full of the right nutrition if they want the best body, but they are not always entirely sure where to begin. Nutrients appear to be somewhat mysterious and a little complex but, in all honesty, they are not. Provided you start from the top and work downwards, nutrients are very simple to understand.

Much of the confusion seems to come from people who say that you "must do it this way" or "you should be eating this and not that." Much of what you hear ends up causing confusion, and nothing seems to fit, making it very difficult to see the big picture. This is why I am going to show you the big picture and let you sort out your own nutrition to meet the goals that you have set. The more time you save for all these, the more time you can spend on other tasks. Knowing that meal preparation and cooking activities are tedious and time-consuming, with the meal prep, you can just buy supplies in bulk, cook once or twice a week, and then you can enjoy the whole week free from kitchen stress. Always remember, meal prepping will help you have a plan. And when you have a plan, you are on the right path to succeed!

Meal Prep for Weight Loss

A Practical Guide For Loosing Extra Kilograms. Stay Concentrated, Feel Better By Weakly Meal Planning. Learn About Fasting, Transformation Techniques and Healthy Nutrition.

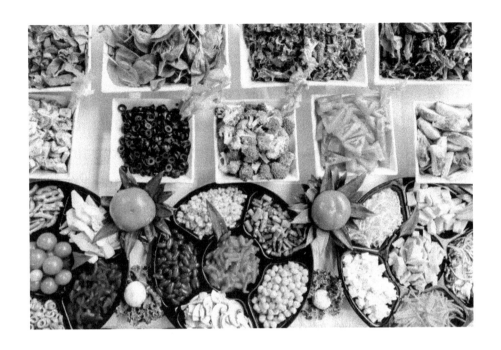

Introduction

Meal prep is in excess of a nourishment pattern: It's a convenient methodology you can use to make heavenly, hand crafted nourishment you'll need to eat each day — without the pause. And keeping in mind that the final products look amazing, meal prep doesn't require confused arranging or devices. All you truly need is time and real effort.

This manual for meal prep shows you all that you have to think about make-ahead meals — in addition to Bulletproof-accommodating methodologies you can take to guarantee your nourishment remains new and nutritious. No nourishment is taboo when you pursue this arrangement, which doesn't make you purchase any prepackaged suppers.

Rapid Weight Loss appoints different nourishments Point esteem. Nutritious nourishments that top you off have less focuses than garbage with void calories. You'll have a Point focus on that is set up dependent on your body and objectives. For whatever length of time that you remain inside your everyday target, you can spend those Points anyway you'd like, even on liquor or treat, or spare them to utilize one more day.

Rapid Weight Loss is intended to make it simpler to change your propensities long haul, and it's adaptable enough that you ought to have the option to adjust it to your life. You'll change your eating and lifestyle designs - a considerable lot of which you may have had for quite a long time - and you'll make new ones.

But now you will have a good solution for your overweight! With this amazing Meal Prep Cookbook, you will easily cut your weight in few weeks. All you need to do is just to follow it and put it into action!

This meal prep cookbook is your answer to fully understanding how to fuel your body so you can burn fat 24/7.

We have prepared with delicious and easy recipes, including: breakfasts, lunches, dinners, that are tasty, delicious. Meantime all recipes include all the macros to make tracking simple. You can find delicious and healthy recipes. With the detailed step by step procedure for each recipe, even the non-cook can prepare these recipes quickly and easily!

Having the macros counted will simplify your life. You will always have an idea of your caloric intake and customize them to your requirements. Most of the recipes can be made in 20 minutes, sometimes less. It will save you too much time! With this amazing fat loss meal prep book, you will achieve incredible effects. In the next few weeks you will be surprised when you stand before the mirror.

Chapter 1   Advantages of Healthy Eating

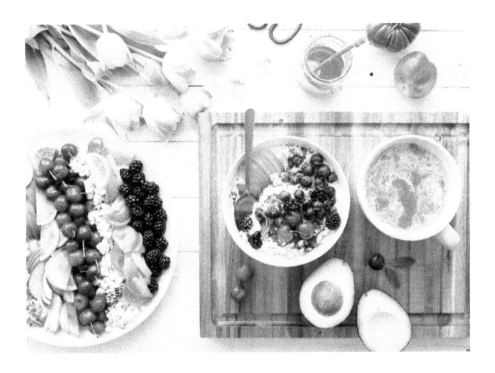

The advantages of healthy eating are countless. Most of us take our bodies for granted. The human body is amazing and is always performing a task. Weather, it is physical, mental or emotional it is always working. Consider healthy eating as a "thank you" to your body. Thank you for all that you do for me on a daily. Be grateful you get to wake up and have one more day with your loved ones. Feeding the body right is more than, just eating the right food. It is also, choosing portion control to limit the weight gain. Fueling our bodies with good nutritious food will help our bodies function efficiently. The body is made up of 70% water. In order for our bodies to not feel muscle aches (due to dehydration), stay "regular," fight off fatigue and illnesses it needs water. Not, soda, coffee or tea but, good ole fashion water.

Most of us don't get enough of it so we are tired, constipated, and sick for most of the winter. Keeping the body hydrated and full of healthy food will dramatically improve the function of the body. Think of your body as a car. I know it seems silly but, stick with me. If you put diesel fuel in a car that takes regular gas what do you think will happen? Yep, the car will have a hard time performing at its best or at all. But, if you put regular gas in it, smooth sailing it will be. Make sense? Now, back to the body. You need "fuel" not just food to keep the body running at its best. The body is designed to eat food that is from the earth, not a lab. Getting healthy isn't easy because you will be changing everything you know and do around food.

Your relationship with food

The relationship you have with food is a big part of how you will lose weight. What are you willing to do to be healthy? That is the question you need to ask yourself.

Find your WHY. Why do you want this? Why are you willing to make the hard changes that need to be made? Once you find you are why that reason will fuel you to keep going and start living a healthy lifestyle. This includes healthy eating, daily exercise, and fueling your mind with positive thoughts and ideas along with getting enough sleep. Keep going even when the goal weight has been achieved. When you get started and see the awesome results you are getting you will not want to give up this lifestyle. You will continue to grow and live a healthy life. One factor that most people overlook is the importance of a good night's sleep. Studies have shown that sleep can actually help you lose weight. Your body needs to rest to reset itself. As we sleep, this is when the body goes to work repairing what has been done throughout the day. The body releases growth hormones to repair tissues that were damaged during the day. Most of the work is done during deep sleep but, if enough sleep isn't happening then, this could lead to other health problems. So, make sure you get your shut-eye is also, very important for your healthy living lifestyle.

In order for us to live a long and healthy life, we need to change our diets and the mind. It needs to consist of lean meats, vegetables, fruits, and LOTS of water. We

can still have junk food but, maybe not as often. Keep
it a balance. Having healthy eating habits doesn't mean
you totally give up the cookies and cake. Yes, you can
have both but, eat junk food in moderation. That is the
beauty of healthy eating. You eat healthy all week and
you still get cake at your grandmother's 80th birthday
party this weekend without feeling guilty about it. It is
a win-win situation all around. It also means keeping
your mindset in check. Meaning, taking care of your
mind as well as your body. The mind is a part of the
body, right? It's a total package and you have to take
care of it all. It will work together and more efficient
getting them on the same page.

Eating healthy can help you maintain a healthy weight,
or it will help you, lose weight by eating less of the junk
and more of the healthy good stuff. Either way, eating
healthy will improve your life on so many levels. The
cravings will come, and you can work through them. If
you are concerned that healthy eating will not taste
good you are wrong. Once, you start to eat healthy on
a regular base the processed food will not taste as good
as it once had. The craving for this food will decrease
and the craving for healthier foods will increase.

There may be times when you eat processed food and
physically feel ill from eating it. It is what your body

gets accustom too. Fight through the urge when the craving monster strikes and just know it will get better each day. Healthy eating will change your physical appearance but, in doing so it will change how you think about yourself and how you see the world. It is almost like magic how one day you wake up and feel different about life. The depression and anxiety will ease if not, disappear altogether. Once you have fuel for the body instead of just food, then it starts to function properly, and you start to feel good! You start to feel better and energy levels go up and that leads to doing more and getting more out of life. Feeling confident in your appearance and fitting into clothes that are a smaller size is such an incredible feeling. You can't help but, have a positive outlook on life and the world. Feeling good will help you look at your stress differently. Things that had stressed you out before may not bother you at all now.

Along with a healthy diet, you should consider an exercise program. Eating healthy alone will not get you the results you are looking for. Healthy eating is the biggest and most challenging part of the whole health journey. Once you get that part of it, the rest is easy. Just because it is hard, shouldn't scare you away from doing it. It's just a challenge at first because you have not done it before. Again, once you understand the concept of it, your life will be more organized than ever before. Well, you're eating habits will be at least.

Healthy eating and the gut

One of the main things you will notice with eating healthy is your gut. If you have stomach issues such as Irritable Bowel Syndrome eating healthy may help ease the pain of that. We were made to eat REAL FOOD! The more we eat the real food the better we will feel as a whole. Eating the food, we were made to eat, will help ease the discomforts processed foods may cause on our stomach. When we eat too much of the processed food our bodies have a hard time breaking it down. So, now bloating, cramping, and just a bad feeling all over, come in to disrupt our busy lives. Protect the gut to eat real food.

When eating healthy it also affects your mind. If you think about all the healthy people you know. Are they negative, sad people? The majority of them are not. They are happy and positive people because they feel good! Feeling happy makes you a more positive person. It goes hand in hand. Positive thinking and feeling good. You start to look at things and your life differently, more positive. You attract happy people because you are feeling that way. You start to understand and question yourself about why didn't I start this sooner? Chemicals in your body are responsible for the "happy" feelings. Endorphin, oxytocin, serotonin, and dopamine.

These chemicals are released when you are feeling good about yourself and how life is going. This brings confidence and pride in your life. When you exercise these chemicals are released into the bloodstream and the mood will be better after the workout. Not only will your thinking become more positive but, fueling the brain is more important because it controls everything in the body. If the brain is running on a low level of nutritional food, it will feel like being in a fog. Studies have shown that people who are obese or diabetic are more likely to develop Alzheimer's disease later in life. Keeping the mind active and continuous learning is another way to keep Alzheimer's at bay studies have shown.

More studies are popping up to show links between what we eat and how our moods are. Nutritional psychology is the science of how nutrients affect mood and behavior. This science is considerably new but, the results that are found are very helpful to the psychology world. Consider treating depression with food instead of drugs. Changing the way, we eat and fuel our bodies could be the best medicine. Once the healthy eating has become the norm, your energy levels will go up and you will have a new outlook on life and stress levels will reduce. This is not a magic solution to all your problems by no means but, healthy eating can reduce stress in your life.

Once you start to feel good, lose weight and feel more confident in yourself the stress you felt about your weight will subside and you will start to feel more positive in your mindset. Things that caused you to feel stressed out before will not seem as bad now that you are feeling good. It all comes back to getting the body and mind aligned. Getting it, all working on the same page. Eating healthy alone isn't going to make you reach your healthy goal weight BUT, it plays a big part in it. If you decide to eat healthy, feed your mind with positive thoughts and expand your awareness, exercise regularly, then you will change inside and out. It is inevitable.

Finding the motivation for healthy eating

Another thing to think about is why do you want this? What are you wanting to change and why? Your way shouldn't be because it is January and everyone else is doing it around me. That will not last and by March you will be done with the whole things. Don't get on the bandwagon and just MAKE yourself do all this change. If you are not mentally ready for the changes believe me they will not come. It doesn't matter how hard you try or how much you suffer eating kale the weight will not come off and all of this will not stick. So, sit down and really think about why you want the changes. It is ok, to take your time and it may take a few days or a week but, you're why should make you cry. Cry because you want this so bad and are willing to try anything to get you to the goal you are setting for yourself. Once you have your WHY then, it is easier to get started and stay committed.

Here is what I mean. Ask yourself why you want to be healthier. Why put yourself through all this change and hard work? Is it because of your kids? You're getting married next year and want to be proud of the wedding pictures that will last forever. Maybe, you are just tired of waking up and hurting in your bones and being uncomfortable with your current situation. Whatever the reason is, write it down and place it where you will see it every day. Physically write in your own handwriting the reason why you want to live a healthier life. Place it on your mirror in the bathroom. Place it in the fridge in the kitchen. Have it on your computer at work. Put it as your screensaver on your phone. Make sure you are seeing it all day every day.

You have to want it for yourself as well. It may start out that you want to be there for your child's graduation from college. At some point, you have to want it for you. You want the change to change you inside and out. Keep a journal of this journey. Write down good days and bad days. Fears and victories. How you are feeling and what you see the future being by you doing this change. This road isn't going to be easy but, it will be worth every blood, sweat, and tear. I hope this book brings the help you need to get started and stick with it. This part may not seem important but, it is. You will be able to look back and see how hard it was and how much stronger you have become mentally and physically. Don't skip this part or just half-ass it. Writing it out and getting it out of your head will make space for more positive thoughts and actions. Besides, writing will help you see how far you have come.

Find a support group or person. Facebook is full of groups that are ready to help you on your journey. It doesn't matter where you are on that journey either. Someone else can help you through the tough times and give you advice on how to navigate through most of it. Support, while changing is so important. You need that person or persons to be accountable when you are not feeling like exercising or eating healthy. They help you stay on track. This person has to give you tough love. They need to tell you to go for that walk and not just tell you it's ok to skip the gym today. A true friend knows that's not what you need. They will make you get up and do the thing you said you were going to do to live the life you want to live. Make sure you can do the same for them. Don't let them wimp out either. Stay strong for each other. Lean on that person for support but, also do the same for them. You won't always feel great and ready to go but, when you know someone else is depending on you to exercise with them you feel more obligated to do it. In turn, keeping you and them on track.

If you have a bad day of eating or you don't exercise. Please do not throw in the towel and say you have ruined everything. Each day is a new day to start over. You don't have to wait till Monday to get started back. If you fall off, get back on even if it is a Thursday. Just pick yourself up and keep going. All of this will get easier. Listen to your body, rest when you are sick or extreme fatigue not when you are being lazy. You know the difference. Push yourself to be better than you were yesterday. Don't compare yourself to someone else.

They may be farther along that you; you can't compare yourself when you are starting out to someone who is far more advanced than you are. They also, maybe 20 years younger and possibly have no kids. That is comparing apples and oranges. Two totally different people. Focus on the task at hand. Focus on your progress and your victories. Be happy for others' accomplishments but, don't underestimate yourself. You are strong and you are mighty. Now that we have that out of the way let's get down to business and learn the tools we need to succeed.

The food we consume today has more chemicals than ever before. Over time this alters our systems on so many different levels. It affects the stomach, liver, brain. It may say low calorie but, what are they replacing to make it that way? Yep, chemicals. What chemicals are doing to the body? Over time these chemicals have been deemed as being the key contributing factors to heart ailments, obesity, diabetes and, all associated offshoots. The most commonly used chemicals are food dyes. They are pretty much in everything processed we eat. Research on Red #40 which is used in 90% of the processed food we eat has been linked to carcinogenic which is cancer-causing. The chemicals used in foods are just those chemicals. Be aware of the ingredients that are in the food we eat. Do research on ingredients you can't pronounce. Some of these ingredients are banned in other countries because the research on these chemicals have strong evidence linking hyper-active in children to them but, they are still legal here in the United States. Know what is in your food. We take it for granted that the government is making that a top priority. Small amounts of chemicals in our food might be ok but, what happens when we eat that chemical for extended periods of time?

To reduce the chemicals that we are ingesting each time we eat consider, a healthy option. Buy fruits and vegetables from the farmers market, locally grown fresh foods. Most of these foods will not be sprayed with pesticides or have added chemicals to them. The processed foods have more chemicals and additives that wreak havoc on the body. If at all possible, consume them only at the very least. The point is to have a healthier life, eat the basic foods that are grown from the earth and not created in a lab. Yes, you can still have the processed food but, eat it in moderation.

Health issues to consider

More and more health problems are showing up in young adults. Some issues could be helped or healed completely if, people would simply change their diet. Insomnia, obesity, depression, anxiety all, have been linked to what we eat and drink on a daily. When a large dose of caffeine is ingested it sticks with you long after you have drunk it. 24 hours to be exact.

Within that, 24-hour window many things take place. The blood pressure and heart rate will increase the first 15 to 30 minutes of drinking it. After about an hour the effects will start to subside, the sugar crash will start to kick in and you are right back where you started but, worse. It will take about 5 to 6 hours for about 50% of the caffeine to subside in the bloodstream. It takes an average of 12 hours for the body to remove all caffeine out of the bloodstream. If drank late in the day, you could have trouble sleeping that night. Along with stressing over financial, relationship, work, kids not sleeping just adds to the list of problems you are having, you could feel overwhelmed and stressed.

If you are consuming energy drinks to stay awake during the day but, have trouble sleeping at night consider taking some time off from the drinks and see if you sleep better. Studies show this is becoming a rising problem in young adults.

Sleep deprivation impairs your judgment, attention, concentration, and problem-solving. Sleep deprivation has been the cause of major accidents all over the world. From Exxon oil spill to Navy ship collision. Getting enough sleep is important. Not getting enough sleep can cause health problems that include cardio symptomatic issues, pulmonary thrombosis and transient ischemic attacks of variant degrees and severities.

Over 6,000 deaths happen a year due to being sleepy behind the wheel. Not only does the lack of sleep become dangerous it also, makes you dumb. When the body isn't getting enough sleep, it starts to impair your learning. It will affect your concentration, attention, alertness and problem-solving skills. It also, makes you forgetful. A study in 2009 infers that within our deepest stages of REM sleep, our memories conjoin and process into sharp-wave ripples. These, in turn, are responsible for causing periods of sleep depravity. Sleep deprivation sounds so intense like we are not sleeping at all. But, that's not always the case. It just means we are not getting enough sleep or yes, a person has insomnia.

Insomnia is when you can't fall asleep or you can't stay asleep.

Weight gain could happen because of a lack of sleep. This situation can correlate into rising levels of desire for sugary, fatty quick-fix band-aid foods and snacks. You can alleviate this by getting enough shut-eye to keep the cravings on the wayside. Sleepiness is the cause of some serious health problems, but, it can also be just plain aggravating not getting enough of it. Here are a few tips to try and help you quiet your mind so you can rest easier.

An hour before bed turn off all the electronic devices. The blue light will stimulate the brain. Making it harder for you to get to sleep. Start the process of going to bed before you actually go to bed. Read a book or do other activities that are relaxing. Start to calm the body and get ready for sleep. Set an alarm on your phone that will go off an hour before you plan on going to bed. This will signal your body to start getting into the sleep mode. At times we get busy with wrapping up the day for everyone else but, taking time for yourself is so beneficial for your sleep. So, make YOU a priority. Make sure the bedroom is dark, cool, and quiet. Take all electronic devices out of the room if at all possible. If that isn't an option to place your phone on the other side of the room. Notifications during the night may wake you and you will have the urge to check the phone. If you have an alarm clock, make sure the light is dim, so as not to disturb you.

Meditation before bed will help the mind relax and be in a calm, peaceful state. Not only is meditation a positive internal chakra alignment in your waking hours each day, the same techniques can relax you at day's end. Learning meditation is strange at first. Because you have never done it before, and it is new. Once you start if only 5 minutes a day or 5 minutes in the morning and 5 minutes at night. The benefits are amazing.

YouTube is full of great meditations. Guided meditations would be good to start out with. They will teach you how to do it and then, you can advance to just doing it on your own with or without music. When doing meditation remember there isn't a right or wrong way to do it.

It is what works for you. If you do better and keep a clear mind (not a blank mind you will always have thoughts come in) by a guided session, then keep doing that. A clear mind is when you have a thought and you can let it go like a bubble on the breeze. Keeping your mind healthy and strong is just as important as keeping your body strong and healthy. If your mind is feeling "off" then, you will feel it throughout your body. You won't want to eat well or exercise. So, keep your mind in check. It makes for a more balanced life.

Energy Drinks

Energy drinks have become a popular alternative to soft drinks. The issue of energy drinks is that they are not regulated under "soft drink" regulations. They are labeled under "supplements." The differences mean more caffeine per 12 ounces can be added to them. The energy drink companies can put in double or even triple the amount of caffeine and they are in legal guidelines to do so. Not, only are you drinking empty calories but, you are putting your heart at risk. There have been reported 34 deaths linked to energy drinks or 5-hour energy since 2004. The visits to emergency rooms due to energy drinks have gone up. From 2007 to 2011 the number of visits had doubled. The average soft drink has about 46 milligrams of caffeine. Monster energy drink has a whopping 240 milligrams of caffeine. The issue and what most people don't understand is an energy drink stays in your system for 24 hours. If you are having trouble sleeping at night or staying asleep, it could be from that energy drink you had at 2 o'clock today. Your heart rate is increased but, when it starts being a problem is when it stays increased for a long period of time. After consuming an energy drink about 20 minutes later you are starting to feel your heart race. The "high" kicks in. The heart doesn't beat it actually flutters.

This isn't good for the heart over long periods of time. The energy drink business is a multibillion-dollar industry. Consider your heart health and just leave the energy drinks alone and get more sleep or drink coffee or tea for that midday pick me up. Drinking plenty of water will help with fatigue as well.

One of the most noticeable side effects of eating healthy is your energy. When first changing you're, diet you are going to think this is so not worth it. While the body is getting rid of the old junk and accepting the good stuff you will feel more tired and maybe, even worse than you have before. Don't worry this will pass. The body is working hard at this time to accept all that is going on. Headaches, fatigue, being hungry may all be side effects to this new life. Again, the body is making changes to work better. It will pass.

Once, processed food is out of your system which may take a few weeks at the most, you will start to feel better. The level of your energy will go up and you will wonder where all of this came from. It comes from limiting sugar in your diet. Sugar will give you a burst of energy for a few hours and then, leave you having a two o'clock crash that will be hard to recover from.

The body produces insulin. Insulin is monitored in the pancreas. It regulates the amount of glucose (sugar) in the bloodstream. The body regulates it throughout the day with the food you eat. When you eat, the body produces insulin to carry to the cells through the bloodstream for energy. If there is extra insulin not used throughout the cells the extra goes to the liver to be stored. A few hours go by and you haven't eaten the liver will release this extra insulin to maintain a constant supply to the body cells. When it becomes a problem is when, over-eating occurs, and a bad diet forces the body to start shutting down the insulin-making process or produces too much.

The body needs insulin to fuel the cells. If they are not getting enough problems will start to occur. Too much glucose in your bloodstream can create problems also. You become an at-risk candidate for cardiac illness, thrombosis, circulatory and renal problems and, acute onset retinopathy. These problems will be for the rest of your life. This is why it is so important to eat healthy now. Eating healthy for your life now and for later. It's a balance. You can have the bad but, eating more healthy foods and getting plenty of exercise is the key to maintaining a healthy body.

To help yourself later in life you need to start taking care of yourself now! Now is the time to consider doing all that you want out of life. Do you still want to be driving and going places when your 80? Living on your own taking care of yourself? Then you need to start taking care of your body now! Thinking of the future is just as important as thinking about now. When we are in our 20's we could eat anything we wanted and wouldn't have to worry about a thing, right? Now, that we are in our 40's or older, we can't eat like that. We are grownups, we have to start eating like one. We have to be an example for our kids and family plus, our community.

Chapter 2   What You Should Know About Weight Loss

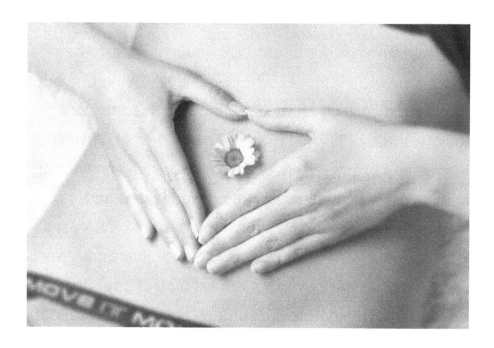

You might need to get more fit for individual reasons. Or on the other hand you may need to get thinner to improve your health. It can decrease your danger of specific issues, similar to coronary illness and type 2 diabetes. It can bring down your circulatory strain and complete cholesterol level. It likewise can assuage side effects and anticipate wounds identified with being overweight.

In any case, there are a few factors that can influence your endeavors to shed pounds. These incorporate making changes to your eating routine, exercise, and lifestyle. There are instruments and tips that can keep you on track. Also, you should recognize what not to do. Converse with your primary care physician before you start another plan. They can assist you with redoing a program and securely screen your advancement. Remember, even little changes can have a major effect in your health.

Way to improved health

Notwithstanding conversing with your primary care physician, there are things you ought to do before you start. You have to focus on the weight-loss plan. Consider advising individuals near you. They can help screen your advance and offer help. This significant demonstration considers you responsible.

When it comes to weight loss, there are 3 significant certainties you should know ahead of time. The first is your weight. The second is your weight file (BMI). Your BMI depends on your weight and tallness. Specialists believe BMI to be the best proportion of your health chance. Truth be told, the medicinal terms "overweight" and "corpulence" depend on the BMI scale. A BMI of somewhere in the range of 25 and 30 is viewed as overweight. A BMI of more than 30 is viewed as corpulent. The higher your BMI, the more prominent your danger of a weight-related ailment. This incorporates type 2 diabetes and coronary illness. Your PCP can help get your BMI, or you can utilize a BMI number cruncher. The BMI diagram is the equivalent for male and female grown-ups. There is a different outline for young ladies and young men under 20 years old. There is additionally a different BMI number cruncher for Asian patients.

The third certainty to know for weight loss is midriff boundary. Muscle versus fat often gathers in your stomach zone. This is all the more a health hazard than muscle versus fat that develops in your thighs or bottom. Thus, your midsection circuit is a significant apparatus. To start, place one finish of a measuring tape over your hipbone. Fold the opposite end over your stomach, ensuring it's straight. The tape shouldn't be excessively tight or too lose.

Specialists believe 40 crawls to be unreasonably high for men and 35 inches unreasonably high for ladies. A high abdomen periphery is known as stomach heftiness. It very well may be an indication of metabolic disorder. This is a gathering of conditions that builds your danger of a weight-related disease. It can prompt sort 2 diabetes or coronary illness.

When you have estimations, set objectives that are down to earth and safe. Your primary care physician additionally can help with this. Your objectives ought to be specific. Be set up for mishaps, yet don't surrender. Prize yourself with something healthy when you hit an objective. For instance, you could attempt another movement, get a back rub, or purchase another outfit. These endeavors will assist you with continuing onward.

Nourishment

All in all, you have to eat less calories than your body utilizes so as to get more fit. Calories originate from the nourishments you eat and drink. A few nourishments have a bigger number of calories than others. For instance, nourishments that are high in fat and sugar are high in calories, as well. A few nourishments are comprised of "void calories." These add a great deal of calories to your eating routine without giving healthy benefit.

If you eat a greater number of calories than your body utilizes, your body stores them as fat. One pound of fat is around 3,500 calories. To lose 1 pound of fat in seven days, you need to eat 3,500 less calories. That partitions out to 500 less calories daily. One thing you can do is expel ordinary soft drink from your eating regimen. This by itself cuts more than 350 calories for every day. You likewise can consume off 3,500 additional calories seven days. You can do this by practicing or being progressively dynamic. The vast majority do a mix of the two. If you do this for 7 days, you can lose 1 pound of fat in seven days.

Most specialists accept that you ought not lose multiple pounds every week. This can imply that you are losing water weight and fit bulk rather than put away fat. It can leave you with less vitality and cause you to recover the weight.

Take a stab at taking a nourishment propensities study. It will disclose to you where you have to make changes to your eating regimen. It likewise can identify what supplements you need. Tips for improving your eating regimen include:

Possibly eat when you are eager. This could mean 3 meals and 1 nibble each day. Or on the other hand it might mean 5 to 6 little meals for the duration of the day. If you aren't ravenous, don't eat.

Try not to skip meals. Skipping meals deliberately doesn't prompt weight loss. It can make you feel hungrier later on. It could make you indulge or settle on poor nourishment decisions.

Hold up 15 minutes before getting a second aiding of nourishment. It can take this long for your body to process whether it's as yet ravenous.

Attempt to eat an assortment of entire nourishments. This incorporates lean meats, entire grains, and dairy. When picking products of the soil, eat the rainbow. Stay away from prepared nourishments and nourishments high in fat or sugar.

Drink a lot of liquids. Pick no-or low-calorie drinks, similar to water or unsweetened tea.

At times, your primary care physician may allude you to a nourishment expert. They can assist you with shopping for food and plans that fit your needs.

Exercise

The two grown-ups and youngsters ought to get customary physical action. It is significant for getting thinner and keeping up great health. The following are approaches to expand your movement and consume calories.

Add 10 minutes every day to your present exercise schedule.

Challenge yourself. Move from moderate to extreme exercises.

Take the stairs rather than the lift.

Park further away or stroll to your goal as opposed to driving.

Accomplish more family tasks, for example, tidying, vacuuming, or weeding.

Take a walk or run with your pooch and additionally kids.

Exercise at home while sitting in front of the TV.

Be dynamic on your excursions. Take a stab at going for a climb or bicycle ride.

Purchase a pedometer or movement tracker. This estimates what number of steps you take every day. Attempt to expand your everyday number of steps after some time. (You can purchase pedometers at outdoor supplies stores.) Some specialists prescribe strolling at any rate 10,000 stages per day.

Point of confinement time spent internet, sitting in front of the TV, and playing computer games. This should approach under 2 hours absolute for each day.

*Average calories consumed for an individual who weighs 154 lbs. If you gauge more, you will consume more calories. If you weigh less, you will consume less calories.

Lifestyle

You may need to modify your calendar to make changes to your eating routine and exercise. This could mean getting up ahead of schedule to work out or preparing your lunch so you don't eat inexpensive food. Alongside diet and exercise, you should make other lifestyle changes. Getting enough rest can assist you with shedding pounds. Rest influences your body's hormones. This incorporates the hormones that tell your body if it is eager or full. You likewise should attempt to decrease your anxiety. Many individuals relate worry to weight gain.

Interesting points

When you start a weight loss plan, there are things to remember. You may have an obstruction that makes it difficult to shed pounds. Or on the other hand it could have led to weight gain in any case. You likewise should be cautious about where you get exhortation. Your weight loss plan ought to be protected and fruitful.

Impediments

The vast majority who are attempting to get in shape have at least one obstruction. You could have unfortunate propensities that began at a youthful age. Propensities are difficult to break, yet they are conceivable. Your PCP can assist you with making transforms, slowly and carefully.

For others, weight addition can be identified with hereditary qualities. You may have a health condition that makes it difficult to shed pounds. Instances of this include:

Hormonal issue

Cushing's infection

Diabetes

Hypothyroidism

Polycystic ovarian disorder (PCOS)

Cardiovascular infections

Congestive coronary illness

Heart valve issue

Idiopathic hypertrophic cardiomyopathy

Rest issue

Obstructive rest apnea

Upper aviation route respiratory disorder

Dietary problems

Bulimia

Sugar longing for disorder.

Certain prescriptions additionally can meddle with your weight loss endeavors. This incorporates:

- Antihistamines for sensitivities
- Alpha or beta blockers for hypertension
- Insulin or sulfonylureas for diabetes
- Progestins for contraception
- Tricyclic antidepressants for wretchedness
- Lithium for hyper wretchedness

- Valproate for epilepsy
- Neuroleptics for schizophrenia.

Converse with your primary care physician about how to deal with your weight regardless of these snags. Lifestyle changes, treatment, or medical procedure can help. You likewise may profit by a care group or guiding.

Diet pills, enhancements, and prevailing fashion consumes less calories

A few organizations and individuals guarantee diet pills cause you to get more fit. This might be valid from the start, yet pills don't assist you with keeping the weight off. They don't show you how to make the essential lifestyle changes. The U.S. Nourishment and Drug Administration (FDA) doesn't test most slim down pills. A significant number of them can have unsafe reactions. Converse with your primary care physician if you think you need an enhancement. They can suggest one that doesn't associate with your medications or conditions. Craze consumes less calories additionally are not demonstrated to be sheltered or assist you with getting more fit. They often offer transient changes, however don't assist you with keeping the weight off. Individuals who advance craze eats less carbs are popular or get paid to make claims. This doesn't make them right or reliable.

There is nobody enchantment diet that enables each individual to get thinner. "Going on an eating regimen" suggests that you will "go off the eating routine" at some point. Try not to depend on a trend diet to take the necessary steps for you. Rather, locate a healthy, adjusted eating plan that can turn into a down to earth lifestyle.

Weight-loss the executives

There are apparatuses you can use all through your weight loss plan. They help to keep tabs on your development and arrive at your objectives.

Regardless of what season it is, there's constantly motivation to drop a couple of pounds.

Now and again, we let ourselves go excessively far and need a major redesign to the manner in which we eat and live. Different occasions, we simply need to fit into that pair of godforsaken pants this month.

In any case, there are a few things to think about weight loss–and our bodies by and large that are basic to see paying little respect to your weight loss objectives.

By understanding these things, your odds of arriving at your objective weight go up and the cerebral pains of grappling with your body to get it to shed some bothersome pounds go down.

Weight loss can change your entire character. That constantly stunned me: Shedding pounds changes your character. It changes your way of thinking of life because you perceive that you are equipped for utilizing your psyche to change your body.

Actualities you have to think about weight loss.

1. Weight is more than fat (center around muscle to fat ratio)

First and in particular, getting that body you need is about something other than weight loss.

Truth be told, weight is excessively broad of a thing to concentrate on if you're extremely genuine about getting fitter because it includes a few elements remembering the measure of muscle for your body and water weight.

Accepting that you're doing a type of solidarity preparing, muscle is pivotal. That is because muscle is heavier than fat, so by losing fat and increasing an identical measure of muscle you'd really be putting on weight. In any case, your body would look slimmer and more slender than at any other time.

2. Drop an inappropriate sort of calories, get enough of the correct ones

Weight loss is about CALORIES. Let's assume it with me, C-A-L... gracious, overlook it. However, it's tied in with turning into an ace at everything calories.

In particular, you have to comprehend what different macronutrients consider calories and what every one does to your body.

Be that as it may, protein and specific sorts of fat are basic for your general health.

The entirety of the above consider calories when devoured, however the difference in your eating routine and weight loss results–can be colossal relying upon what number of every you expend.

3. Track your nourishment consumption

Moving off of the last point, you have to begin viewing your nourishment consumption like you watch for updates on the following period of Stranger Things.

Be that as it may, for the most part, you need to devour simply under your suggested day by day caloric admission. This will make your body start consuming fat with the goal that it can keep up its fundamental vitality utilization level (because it needs to get it from some place and it will go first to your fat store).

4. Rest can really assist you with losing weight. The Science Behind a Good Night's Sleep

As with truly everything else attached to your physical and emotional well-being, rest is basic for weight loss. Rest is a period for everything in the body to revive and upgrade itself, including when the greater part of the fat and general calorie-consuming procedures happen, so by getting enough rest you're giving your body the time it needs to drop those inches.

5. Make healthy nourishment advantageous (and lousy nourishment not)

Weight loss needs to go with lifestyle changes, else, you'll also effectively shift once more into your old examples and come back to your unique weight.

You don't have to free yourself of them altogether. Truth be told, doing so can hurt your weight loss endeavors as you'll see later, yet you do need to lessen the danger of those allurements while improving the probability of picking another healthier alternative.

6. Jettison the scale

Gazing at a scale each day can be out and out dampening. That is because our weight vacillates during each time consistently whether we're attempting to get more fit or not.

Some portion of this is because of the water content in our body, some portion of it the backwards connection between muscle to fat ratio loss and muscle gain, just as other standard substantial vacillations.

Be that as it may, if you truly need to take a gander at the scale, then do it week by week and take a gander at it a couple of times in that day to show signs of improvement normal weight.

7. Weight loss pills are an awful, ill-conceived notion

I know, the possibility of a mystical weight loss pill making your fat break down away like a fantasy is alluring. Yet, oh dear, it's unrealistic (if that wasn't clear as of now).

Here's a thought of a portion of the symptoms of weight loss pills:

Pneumonic hypertension (possibly deadly)

Coronary illness

Increment circulatory strain

Expanded pulse

A sleeping disorder

Dazedness

Anxiety

Weight loss pills often guarantee prompt outcomes. In any case, they don't do anything to change your eating regimen or physical exercise propensities, capacity to oppose enticement, and the various propensities that made your body the weight it is presently. In this way, regardless of whether do figure out how to move beyond the dreadful symptoms and get results, you'll in the end up back where you began.

To make a genuine, enduring change, you have to change your wellness and sustenance propensities.

8. You can't simply continue cutting calories

I comprehend what you may be thinking then. "I need results quick, so I'll simply cut calories definitely and arrive faster."

All things considered, the math essentially includes. Correct? Right?... .

Wrong. Starving yourself with too scarcely any calories is a no-no, so don't consider attempting to quick track your eating routine by eating air. Tragically, it simply doesn't work that way.

10. A cheat day is an absolute necessity (however not for the explanation you're thinking)

You've presumably known about a cheat day prior: a day where, stuck between recollections of a severe, excruciating eating regimen and the fear of a difficult week loaded up with exhausting, lifeless meals, is a shine of expectation that you can devour anything you desire and in whatever amount.

For this one day, you have complete opportunity. Need to get those cupcakes you saw not long ago at the store? Go wild. Dessert? Stack those scoops. Starbucks? Be brave make it a venti.

Be that as it may, what the vast majority aren't mindful of is a cheat day has a completely different and much increasingly basic job in an eating regimen: to keep up metabolic rate.

Stop and think for a minute: your new diet can possibly hinder your digestion because you'll be expending less calories. When this occurs, you'll consume less calories and your weight loss portion will be that a lot harder to hit.

In any case, by having one day in the week where you go wild, you're advising the body that it needs to keep up its current metabolic rate, expanding your weight loss endeavors throughout the entire week and having fun all the while.

11. Meal preparing makes everything simpler

Truly, adhering to a severe eating routine isn't basic for weight loss—it's out and out depleting.

It takes a great deal of work to assemble an eating regimen that can assist you with getting thinner, notwithstanding, it's justified, despite all the trouble. What's more, setting aside the effort to prepare those meals in advance every week makes it exponentially simpler to adhere to that diet because you've evacuated any kind of protection from it, making it simpler just to eat what is now before you instead of going to get or make something different.

12. Use HIIT (and quality preparing)

It's critical to work out if you're extremely genuine about getting thinner, be that as it may, it's sufficiently bad to simply toss on one of those old Jazzercise recordings and get going (as much as I probably am aware you like them).

Research has demonstrated the advantages of HIIT or high-power interim preparing are far more noteworthy than your normal exercise for both cardio and weight preparing, both significant pieces of a total weight loss routine (cardio drops calories and keeps your heart healthy, quality preparing enables consume to fat).

With HIIT, you can get a similar advantage in a short time what you'd get in one hour of an ordinary exercise.

13. Drop the end of the week drinks, couple-starting up discussion drinking-moving

As dismal glad as it may sound to a few, dropping liquor can quickly bring about dropping pounds.

A great many people aren't mindful of exactly what number of calories are in their preferred beverages, now and again significantly more than sugary soft drinks, so by dropping liquor or decreasing your admission, you can gain some truly necessary ground quick.

14. Try not to accuse your thyroid

Growing up, I had a companion with a thyroid issue. She was somewhat powerful as a kid, at the same time, when the issue was found all that abundance weight vanished and never returned.

As promising as this sounds, she's a minority. For the vast majority, ladies being the more typical case, this isn't the issue. What's more, by attempting to search for different reasons why you probably won't be the weight you'd prefer to be, you're simply giving yourself pardons. Be sensible yet additionally be straightforward with yourself.

15. More water, less Starbucks

Notwithstanding liquor, huge numbers of different beverages we expend consistently have gigantic measures of calories. This incorporates:

Pop

Juice

Lattes/comparative Starbucks-like beverages

The thing is, rather than the sorts of important calories we discussed before, similar to protein and great fats, these are vacant calories that essentially top us off and make us put on weight. As such, we needn't bother with them.

Rather, drink bunches of water, which doesn't simply assist you with cutting the calories yet enables your body's different procedures to run easily, which can help aid weight loss.

16. It's less what you're devouring and progressively about over expending

If you think sugar, liquor, gluten, or some other sort of nourishment or drink is making you fat, surmise once more. Certainly, every one of these has an impact, in any case, it's less about what singular things you're expending and increasingly about the amount you're devouring.

Indulging is the thing that outcomes in weight acquire (calories than our body needs to work), so if you cut back on your Starbucks, bring down your liquor utilization, and diminish the occasions you eat at Pepe's in a month, you can keep everything you like while definitely decreasing your carbohydrate content and shedding some weight.

17. Everybody's body is different

This is effectively one of the most significant focuses to remember.

At a certain point or another, we as a whole hear that XYZ big name, companion, or relative did some specific eating regimen that did some incredible things for them.

The thing is, everybody's body is different and there's all the more a probability that equivalent technique won't work for you, so focus on your own body, and find what works for you.

18. There are no speedy fixes. Morning exercise is one of the most dominant approaches to begin your day

There are things you can do to lose a touch of weight rapidly (like dropping liquor), be that as it may, it's imperative to remember that there are zero handy solutions to genuine, significant weight loss.

Try not to pay any mind to any big name prevailing fashion diet, they're simply playing to the restless masses. You should be eager to practice something beyond your body to get more fit. You have to practice your understanding.

19. Make it a lifestyle

The last and conceivably most significant thing of all to know is this: healthy living, regardless of whether it's dropping a couple of pounds now, a great deal of pounds throughout the following year, building muscle, or something different, should be made a lifestyle.

This is more mental than everything else, except it profoundly affects your capacity to stay steady in your exertion, the prime enemy in any undertaking, including getting more fit.

How to Meal Prep for Weight Loss

We've already determined meal prep is a powerful tool to facilitate weight loss, and now it's time to prepare. This chapter is the "how-to" chapter. I'll walk you through preparation so you have everything you need. We will also discuss the practicality of meal prep, including food safety and food storage options.

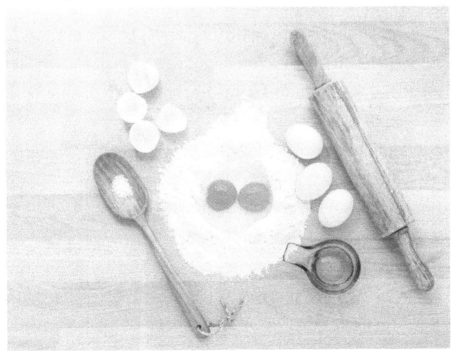

Step-by-Step Weight Loss

With a good meal prep plan, weight loss can be as simple as 1-2-3. You are developing a new skill set that you can never unlearn. By learning all about meal prep and following the steps outlined in this book you will be able to lose weight and keep it off.

SET YOUR TARGET

First, it's a good idea to set your goal for what you want to achieve by meal prepping. I love the acronym S.M.A.R.T. for setting goals. It stands for Specific, Measurable, Attainable, Realistic, and Timely. Using this acronym creates accountability for your goals.

For example, let's turn the generic goal of "weight loss" into a S.M.A.R.T. goal. You might say your goal is to lose 8 pounds by June 1st by meal prepping once a week on Sundays at 10 a.m.

Take a minute to write down your own S.M.A.R.T goal answering these questions:

•How much weight do you want to lose?

•When will you achieve this goal?

•How often will you meal prep?

•When will you meal prep?

WHAT TO EAT?

As mentioned before, we will follow the plate method for creating nutritional balance in our meals. Balanced meals lead to better energy levels, fewer cravings, and sustainable weight loss. This section covers what to fill your meal prep container with to help you lose weight and keep it off—permanently.

Protein stimulates metabolism, balances blood sugar, builds lean tissue, and supports immune function. Include a protein source at every meal, including egg whites, high-protein dairy products (cottage cheese and Greek yogurt), poultry, fish, shellfish, lean beef cuts (like 96 percent lean ground beef), lean pork cuts (like boneless pork chops), lentils, tofu, or edamame.

Produce is abundant in life-sustaining and disease-fighting antioxidants, vitamins, minerals, and phytochemicals. These nutrients are best absorbed from food versus taken as supplements. Produce also provides fiber, which helps keep you fuller longer. Most fiber comes from non-starchy vegetables, which include but are not limited to:

•Artichokes

•Asparagus

•Bean sprouts

•Bell peppers

•Broccoli

•Brussels sprouts

•Cabbage

- Cauliflower
- Celery
- Cucumbers
- Eggplants
- Mushrooms
- Onions
- Peppers
- Salad greens
- Spinach
- Squash (all types: spaghetti, yellow, acorn, delicata, etc.)
- Sweet mini peppers
- Tomatoes
- Turnips
- Zucchini

When it comes to starch and weight loss, both quality and quantity matter. High-quality carbohydrates are those in the least processed form, which have higher levels of filling protein and fiber. Examples include, but are not limited to:

- Barley
- Beans (except lentils and edamame)
- Brown rice
- Corn
- Couscous

- Farro
- Oats
- Peas
- Plantains
- Potatoes
- Quinoa
- Sweet potatoes
- Whole fruit (not fruit juice)
- Whole wheat

Don't fear fat. It is essential to metabolism and function. Your brain is 60 percent fat; hormones are made from fat; and every cell in your body is surrounded by fat. Opt for several servings per day of the following foods:

- Avocados
- Egg yolks
- Fatty fish like salmon and tuna
- Olives
- Organic grass-fed dairy products
- Nuts including peanuts, and seeds

I also recommend cooking with unrefined cold-pressed avocado oil and using olive oil for colder items like salad dressings.

HOW MUCH TO EAT?

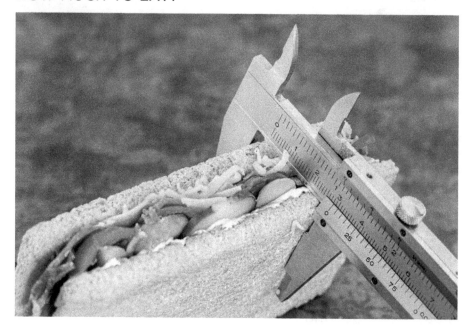

Your overall caloric needs are unique to you, but if you focus on setting up your portions using these guidelines you'll be off to a good start in meeting them. Recipes in the meal plans follow this setup so you'll gain some practice cooking meals that follow this portion guide. Carbohydrates: Some carbohydrates break down into sugar in the body and some carbohydrates are indigestible (fiber), passing through the GI system untouched. Both non-starchy vegetables and starchy vegetables provide carbohydrates. Modify this amount as needed, aiming for about 40 percent of your calories coming from carbohydrates, but not exceeding 45-ish grams per meal. If you are very active (for example, training for a marathon) you may need to increase this amount, up to 65 percent, exceeding the 45 grams per meal guideline. Otherwise, stick with 40 percent.

Aim to get a minimum of 25 grams and 40 grams of fiber, for women and men respectively. Please don't worry about net carbs (total carbs minus fiber); just get in your minimum fiber for the day. That said, there are some recipes in this book that exceed 45 grams of carbs per recipe but not 45 grams of net carbs. Try not to get too caught up or obsessed with the numbers; the ultimate goal is to create balance in each meal and throughout the day.

Non-starchy veggies: Your fists are proportionate to your body, so they are a great way to eyeball portion sizes. Aim for two fistfuls of vegetables at each meal, for at least two meals a day.

Starch: About ½ cup, or 30 to 45 grams, per meal is appropriate for most people trying to lose weight.

Protein: One palm-size (4- to 6-ounce) portion should equal 20 to 30 grams of protein. Most women should get one portion and men should get two portions at each meal.

Healthy fat: Aim for 1 to 2 tablespoons per meal or snack. Fat is calorie dense, so you do need to watch your portions, but it's also filling so don't skip it. Just make sure there is a little healthy fat in the meal either added at the end or during the cooking process.

Drinks: Water, black tea, coffee, infused fruit water, and sparkling water are great options. For weight loss, weight maintenance, and general health, avoid high-sugar beverages such as soda, juice, sports drinks, and other drinks with added sugars.

MAKE YOUR PLAN

To create a meal prep plan, you must first create a quick meal plan.

1.Look in your cabinets and freezer and make a list of things you need to use up.

2.Use the ingredients to plan recipes into your week.

3.Make a list of the recipes you want to prep ahead of time.

4.Make a list of ingredients you don't have that you need to make the recipes you selected.

What I Have   Recipes to Make

    What I Need

SELECTING RECIPES

Almost any recipe can be meal-prep friendly, but there are a few things to keep in mind when selecting recipes to make, such as:

•Does it contain healthy ingredients (free of processed foods)?

•Does it follow the plate method, or can it be modified to follow this method?

•Will the food be easy to store?

•Will the food reheat well? Example: The air fryer craze is fun, but the food doesn't reheat nearly as crispy and tasty as you'd like.

GATHER WHAT YOU NEED

Having some basic kitchen gear will allow you to begin meal prepping with ease. This section outlines the equipment and tools needed for meal prep, and offers some tips to keep grocery costs down.

HELPFUL TOOLS AND EQUIPMENT

Kitchen Equipment

Not a lot is required to begin meal prepping. These kitchen basics will get you started:

•8-by-8-inch casserole dish

•9-by-13-inch casserole dish

•Aluminum foil, heavy-duty

•Baking sheets (2)

•Large nonstick skillet with lid

- Muffin tin with silicone liners or silicone muffin tin
- Oven
- Oven-safe skillet
- Slow cooker
- Stovetop

Meal Prep Equipment

- Airtight storage containers
- Divided airtight storage containers
- Insulated lunch bag for transporting food
- Mason jars and lids

SHOPPING IN BULK

Shopping in bulk is a great way to save money and always be prepared for meal prepping. Freeze unused portions for use in future meal preps. Food items that are great to purchase in bulk are:

- Beans
- Cooking oils
- Fish
- Grains (oats, quinoa, etc.)
- Nuts
- Poultry
- Seeds
- Shellfish

Note: Bulk bins are not suitable for those with food allergies as foods can easily become cross-contaminated with potential allergens.

Throughout the book, I use avocado oil for cooking. Unrefined cold-pressed avocado oil is very stable at high temperatures and has similar health benefits to olive oil. When purchased in bulk, the price point is comparable to olive oil. However, you can substitute canola oil or olive oil for avocado oil in any recipe in this book.

Chickpea flour is a high-protein flour utilized in a few recipes in this book. Whole-wheat flour can be used instead of chickpea flour but, when purchased in bulk, chickpea flour can be very affordable.

For weight loss, my preferred baking flour is almond flour because its fat and protein content is more satiating. You cannot substitute any other flour for almond flour because it is a high-fat, high-protein flour. Almond flour can be purchased in bulk to save money.

Other Ways to Keep Costs Down:

•Avoid purchasing items in bulk that might go bad and can't be frozen, such as dairy.

•Buy beans canned.

•Cook meatless meals one night per week.

•Eat from the pantry (use what you have).

•Freeze unused fruit for smoothies.

•Limit more expensive organic purchases to the EWG Dirty Dozen™ list.

•Shop sales and use coupons.

•Shop seasonal produce.

EXECUTE EFFICIENTLY

The goal of meal prepping is to learn to be as efficient as possible, so you spend the least amount of time in the kitchen, but make the most of it for your healthy eating goals. You will naturally get faster at meal prep the more practice you have. This section provides time-saving tips to get you started.

PLANNING THE COOK SESSION

In general, work from the most time-consuming item to the least. For example:

1. Slow cooker recipes should be started first.
2. Recipes with long cooking times go in the oven next.
3. Sheet pan recipes with shorter cooking times follow.
4. Hands-on stovetop recipes follow.
5. No-bake recipes are completed last.

Decide whether you will do one or two preps per week, then split up the meals accordingly. Depending on the selected recipes and your schedule in a given week, you may choose to do one prep some weeks and two preps per week at other times.

EFFORT-SAVING TIPS AND TRICKS

1.Cook items in bulk that can be used for various meals, such as brown rice, quinoa, or shredded chicken, and freeze the remaining portion for another week.

2.You don't have to cook every single meal for the whole week. Cook ingredients that take time but are components of your selected recipes, like grains, for use in recipes later in the week.

3.If budget allows, purchase already cut and washed produce. You can also use frozen foods to save time on prep work.

4.Repeat meals. Make sure you provide variety from week to week but, during the week, repeat meals as often as possible to save time in the kitchen.

5.Use the same ingredients in multiple recipes.

Chapter 3   Macronutrients

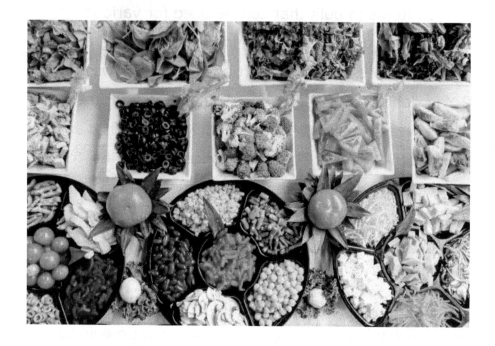

Remember the old food pyramid where the large, sturdy base was made up of bread, cereal, and other carbohydrates, six to eleven servings per day? The next level contained vegetables with three to five servings and fruits with two to four servings. Then, higher up but with smaller servings required are the dairy, meat, egg, nuts, and beans with two to three servings. This was all crowned by fats, oils, and sweets at the tip top. There are no serving suggestions but a warning that said: "USE SPARINGLY."

These guidelines sounded reasonable and made sense with what we knew about the body's use of nutrition. But, what the food pyramid didn't take into account is that most foods contain some carbs, protein, and fat. Our bodies need a balance of these nutrients to function efficiently by burning unwanted fat but not running out of energy.

Because of that first introduction to the basic food groups, there is a tendency to think of bread as strictly carbohydrate. Vegetables, fruits, and foods at the same level are thought of as health food. In other words, you can eat them as much as you want, while most types of meat, dairy, eggs, and nuts are good-for-you protein. On top of the pyramid is fat. "So, who eats a stick of butter? I shouldn't have a problem with fat!"

Fortunately, food science and our understanding of how we break down the components of food have come a long way since the first attempt to help people eat healthily. The old version of the food pyramid laid the groundwork for a variety of new views. Diets such as Paleo, Atkins, Keto, and others are formulated around increasing or decreasing the intake of carbs, proteins, and fats.

It turns out that those three main elements of carbohydrates, proteins, and fats are the three major nutrients contained in the food we eat. *They are called macronutrients* or macros for short.

Macros: The Building Blocks of Food

We have to re-learn the way we think of food. Instead of thinking of bread as a carb, an apple as "health food," an egg as protein, or walnut as fat, we look at the percentage of all three macros in the food. What percentage of carbs, protein, and fat do the bread, apple, egg, and walnut contain?

It sounds complicated, but it really isn't. The percentages are conveniently contained on the product's nutrition label. For whole foods such as avocado or spaghetti squash, there are online nutrient calculators that you can use to figure the percentage spread.

Are you feeling overwhelmed? Don't be. By the time you finish these, you will be a pro at figuring your macro percentages needed to reach your goals. You will also have the tools you need to find the proper food to fuel your body.

A Closer Look at Macronutrients

1. Carbohydrates:

You have probably heard about simple and complex carbohydrates. Here is a definition refresher.

Simple carbs break down fast and are absorbed quickly into the bloodstream. Some foods that are considered simple carbs are: *refined sugar, fruit juice, candy, honey, white potatoes, white rice, refined white flour, alcohol, syrups, and sodas*.

Complex carbs, on the other hand, are released slowly in the bloodstream over some time to help sustain your body's energy. Some foods that are considered complex carbs are: quinoa, brown rice, beans, lentils, oatmeal, and peas.

Are you familiar with the term sugar rush? That's what happens when your energy slumps, and you feel tired, so you eat a simple carb (say, a chocolate bar) to give you quick energy. Unfortunately, this quick fix of energy burns out as fast as it peaks. Then, you experience a sugar crash, which leaves you feeling worse than before.

Layering complex carbs with simple carbs is a better use of this nutritional building block. Cyclist will carbo-load with whole grains and other complex carbs several days before a big ride so that they have an extra store of energy (glycogen) in the muscles and liver. This prevents the athlete from running out of energy before finishing the race.

During the race, the athlete can consume some simple carbs to give him or her an extra boost of energy. This is not harmful because the athlete is burning up calories at an amazing rate.

For those of us sitting and watching the race, we don't need that sugary drink or sweet snack. Unfortunately, we are not burning many calories as we cheer on the riders.

Beware of cutting too many carbs out of your diet. If the body does not have enough carbohydrate to convert into glucose, it will start using protein and fat to do this process. This method of creating glucose has a waste product called ketones that build up in the body, causing the kidneys to work extra hard to clear out the waste.

The fiber in carbohydrates plays an important role in the health and welfare of your body. Keeping your bowel movements regular is what fiber is best known for, but dietary fiber appears to have a much more important role. High-fiber diets appear to lower risk of heart disease, high blood pressure, diabetes, and obesity.

2. Protein:

Protein is not stored in the body but is found in almost every part of the body, nails, hair, skin, bone, muscle, and tissue.

Proteins are made up of more than twenty different amino acids, nine of which are essential and must come from the food you eat. The body gets these amino acids in one of two ways: building them from scratch or modifying others. Foods called *high-quality proteins* such as dairy products, meat, and eggs, have all the essential amino acids that the body requires.

Compare red meat, ham steak, grilled salmon, chicken, and lentils/beans. Take into account fat and salt content. You will find that protein from dairy (whey), grilled fish, some chicken and lentils/beans are the best option to lower saturated fats and sodium.

And, you can do the environment some good by cutting down on red meat as the methane gas created by all those cows contributes to the greenhouse effect. Greenhouse gas emissions by cattle as a natural part of their digestive process and how we deal with the manure help contribute to the buildup of greenhouse gases in our atmosphere.

3. Fat:

Saturated Fats — Animal fats such as lard (bacon fat) and dairy fats (butter, cheese) and anything hard at room temperature contains saturated fat. You also need to steer clear of some tropical oils such as palm and palm kernel and coconut.

Trans Fats — Stay away from these manufactured fats that are created by hydrogenating oils (forcing extra hydrogen atoms onto a fat chain hardens the oils). If you see partially hydrogenated oil on the food label, that is code for trans fats. Try to avoid eating this product.

Unsaturated Fats

Monounsaturated fats

Polyunsaturated fats

Omega-6 fatty acids

Calorie Counting vs. Macro Counting

What is the difference between counting calories and counting macros? When we count calories, we are counting the number of calories (energy) we consume from the food regardless of the nutrient source. When counting macros, we count the calories consumed from each of the nutrients.

This is the calculation you need to remember to find out where your calories come from:

- One gram of carbs = 4 calories
- One gram of protein = 4 calories
- One gram of fat = 9 calories

The basic ratio your body needs per day is 30% carbs, 40% protein, and 30% fat. Now, this can change depending on your personal health goals that you have set up with your physician.

For example, the average slice of whole grain with seed bread has about 120 calories per slice listed on the food label. So that's 120 calories used up from our daily allotted amount. But in terms of macros we read: carbs 22g, protein 5g, and fats 2g.

Using our calories per gram formula above, we do the following:

- 22g of carbs * 4 calories = 88 calories from carbs
- 5g of protein * 4 calories = 20 calories from protein
- 2 grams of fat * 9 calories = 18 calories from fat
- Giving: 88 + 20 + 18 = 126 calories per slice.

Again, using an online fitness tool with a built-in nutrition calculator makes tracking your intake much easier. For your convenience, there is a page at the back of the book for manual tracking to get you started and a list of sites that provide online calculators.

Male: 55, 5' 11", current weight 185, goal weight 170. Lightly active (moderate exercise by sedentary job). This person wants to lose fifteen pounds.

Using the online Macronutrient Calculator from *www.bodybuilding.com*, the daily macros needed to lose weight at a moderate pace would be 168 g carbs, 168 g protein, and 37 g fats per day. Taking this one step further:

- 168g * 4c = 672 carbs
- 168g * 4c = 672 protein
- 37g * 9c = 333 fat
- Giving: 672+672+333= 1677 calories per day

Using the online calorie calculator from *www.freedieting.com*, I find that: maintenance is 2335 cals per day, fat loss is 1868 cals per day, and extreme fat loss is 1480 cals per day.

Because we do not know exactly how these sites are creating their numbers, talk to your doctor in order to find out what calories per day is best for your weight goal.

Using calories of 1868 per day in the macro calculator, the macro ratio comes to 40% carbs, 30% protein, and 30% fat.

Grams per day = 186g carbs, 140g protein, and 62g fat.

- 186g * 4c = 744 carb
- 140g * 4c = 560 protein
- 62g * 9c = 558
- Giving: 744+560+558 = 1862 cals per day.

Putting This Information to Use

Sex: M

Weight: 190

Height: 5' 11"

Exercise: 3 times a week, 30 minutes

Job: Sedentary

Goal Weight: 170, loss of 20 lbs

Maintain: 2138 calories

Moderate Fat Loss: 1710 calories

Extreme Fat Loss: 1520 calories

Sex: F

Weight: 170

Height: 5' 4"

Exercise: 3 times a week, 30 minutes

Job: Sedentary

Goal Weight: 150, loss of 20 lbs

Maintain: 1860 calories

Moderate Fat Loss: 1488 calories

Extreme Fat Loss: 1360 calories

Using several well-established restaurants and their online nutritional information, I came up with an example of what might be a typical meal plan for the average American.

Brea kfast	Table 1	gCa rbs	gPr ot	gFa t		cCar bs	cPr ot	cFa t	Calories
	2 Scrambled	2	15	17		8	60	153	221
	Whole Grain Toast with butter, jam	58	7	11		232	28	99	359
	Hash Browns	19	2	14		76	8	126	210
	Bacon, 2 slices	1	7	7		4	28	63	95
Lunc h	SW Chicken Club	43	29	29		172	116	261	549
Dinn er	Meatloaf with mashed potatoes and broccoli	92	44	42		368	176	378	922
Daily Total s		215	104	120		860	416	108 0	2356

As you can see in Table 1, one size does not fit all. Both male and female are over the maintenance range, but the female is way over. This may be part of the reason that women have a bigger struggle with weight loss. Portions are geared toward larger bodies with bigger appetites. Combine large portions of high fat and carb options with our eating on-the-fly American lifestyle, and you have a recipe for obesity.

Look for ways you can change your meal to better fit your new habits. Order the eggs poached or basted (cooked in water or steamed). Eat one slice of toast and have it dry (no butter or jam). Or, make sure you order the toast dry so that you can control how much fat and sugar you add. Skip the hash browns altogether, or see if they have a fresh fruit option. Bacon was a better choice than sausage, so no change is needed.

The easiest change for lunch and supper is to cut the order in half. Order half a sub, or better yet, make it veggie with grilled chicken, vinegar only, and no oil. With the dinner, ask for a to-go box, and put half aside for lunch tomorrow. You can look at the grid above to see how much you save by cutting things in half and leaving off the extras.

Let's look at some more information that needs to be taken into account when trying to improve our eating habits.

Using Food Labels: Measures and Weights

One of the best laws our government ever passed for the people of the United States is Public Law 101-535, which is the Nutrition Labeling and Education Act (NLEA).

President George H. W. Bush signed the act into law on November 8, 1990.

This law gives the FDA (Food and Drug Administration) authority to require nutrition labels on almost everything we eat. Over the past 30 years, the label contents have been enhanced to include valuable information for consumers.

Let's take a look at a label to see what information is included.

Nutrition Facts

Serving Size 1 cup (228g)
Servings Per Container 2

Amount Per Serving

Calories 250   Calories from Fat 110

	% Daily Value*
Total Fat 12g	**18%**
Saturated Fat 3g	**15%**
Trans Fat 3g	
Cholesterol 30mg	**10%**
Sodium 470mg	**20%**
Potassium 700mg	**20%**
Total Carbohydrate 31g	**10%**
Dietary Fiber 0g	**0%**
Sugars 5g	
Protein 5g	
Vitamin A	**4%**
Vitamin C	**2%**
Calcium	**20%**
Iron	**4%**

* Percent Daily Values are based on a 2,000 calorie diet. Your Daily Values may be higher or lower depending on your calorie needs.

	Calories:	2,000	2,500
Total Fat	Less than	65g	80g
Sat Fat	Less than	20g	25g
Cholesterol	Less than	300mg	300mg
Sodium	Less than	2,400mg	2,400mg
Total Carbohydrate		300g	375g
Dietary Fiber		25g	30g

Start here

Check calories

Quick guide to % DV

5% or less is low
20% or more is high

Limit these

Get enough of these

Footnote

Using a bread label for this example, **Nutrition Facts** heads the familiar column of information.

First up is the **Serving Size** listed in standard units, followed by metric units, and then **Servings Per Container**. Pay attention to serving size. Some bread labels are 1 slice, some 2 slices. You can torpedo all your hard work if you think you are logging macros for 2 slices when it was actually 1 slice serving.

Serving information is always followed by **Calories** per serving and **Calories from Fat**. Try to steer clear of food that has more than 50% of calories from fat. One exception would be avocado, which is high in fat but no saturated or trans fats. This is an example of a food that has fats necessary for hormone production and cell maintenance.

In the next block of the label, we find the nutrients, including the macros. The nutrients are listed in metric along with the percentage based on the daily requirement of 2000 calories. Here, you will find **Total Fat** broken down by **Saturated Fat** and **Trans Fat**. **Cholesterol, Sodium, Potassium** are listed next and are especially important to people with diabetes, high blood pressure, and other life-threatening diseases. **Total Carbohydrates** is broken down into **Dietary Fiber** and **Sugars**. Items high in dietary fiber are a much better choice than those with high sugar numbers (sometimes added) and little or no dietary fiber. The last item in the nutrients is **Protein**.

The next block of the label list **trace vitamins and minerals** contained in the product. These listings come in handy when you are trying to increase or limit a certain vitamin or mineral. For example, if you are on a medication that requires a low vitamin K diet, this is the place on the label you would check for the percentage of daily requirements of vitamin K this serving of food fulfills.

The final block of the label is an explanation of the minimum daily requirements based on a 2000 calorie diet and sometimes, a 2500 calorie diet.

Don't forget to check the *ingredients list* that usually follows the nutrition label. If you are purchasing something that claims to be made with chicken, is chicken the first ingredient? If not, do you really want to eat that product?

Also, if the ingredients list contains "partially hydrogenated ...," skip this item. That means that the product contains trans fats, and you do not want to add those to your diet.

How Do Carb/Protein/Fat Work in the Body?

Macronutrients are the three building blocks of food that your body need to thrive, but how do carbs, protein, and fats work to fuel your body?

Carbohydrates — Both simple and complex carbs are converted into energy by the body in the form of glucose, the main source of energy for the body. Though, as we saw above, complex carbs do a better job of giving us a steady flow of energy.

Carbs also benefit the body in other ways. The fiber found in many carbs helps clean our bowels and appear to help with some health issues, such as reducing high blood pressure, diabetes, and obesity.

Protein — Made of components called amino acids, protein is in charge of growth and tissue repair. A quick reminder: there are 20 different amino acids. Eleven of these, we produce with our bodies, and nine essentials must be obtained from the food we eat.

Fat — The macronutrient fat has its share of important functions. We think of it mainly as a means of storing excess energy—in the form of fat. But, it is also instrumental in absorbing the fat-soluble vitamins (A, D, E and K), which are used in the production of some hormones and help with maintaining cell structures.

Setting Weight Goals

This is where meal planning really helps. As you can see above, the amount of food and what the meal consists of are extremely important.

To give meal planning a chance, you need to set up your food intake to match the outcome desired. Take your weight prior to starting the three weeks. Leave the scales alone during your first three weeks on the plan, then check the results. I'm guessing you really won't be surprised, because your clothes will fit better or feel a bit loose, and you'll be feeling better.

Using the tools you have been given, work up your meal plan based on your weight loss goals. Then, make an appointment with your doctor to have him or her review the plan with you.

Chapter 4   Meal Planning And Meal Prepping

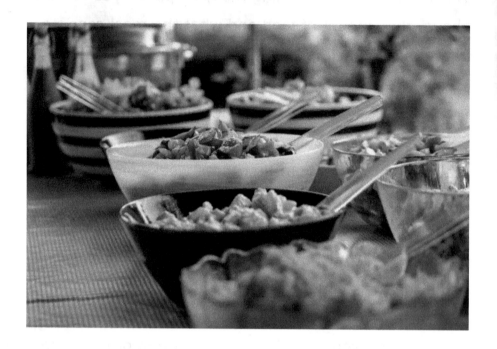

Meal planning

Meal planning is planning what you will eat for the week ahead. It can be for an individual or a family.

Meal prepping

It is simply making your meals ahead of time! So, you don't have to cook day in and day out. What you are doing here is essentially preparing your meals ahead of time and storing these pre-cooked meals in containers. Meal prepping is perfect for people—like you and me—who live busy lives yet still want to have full control over the food we eat and the benefits that we get from whole foods.

Importance of Meal Prep

You can avoid decision fatigue: What am I going to eat today? What is there to eat? Are just some of the few questions you need not to ask yourself on a daily basis when on meal prep. One of the reasons why many people lose your motivation on following the ketogenic diet is that you get tired of figuring out which food is acceptable, and which isn't. When you start to experience decision fatigue, you are prone to grabbing any food that you can find in your pantry or fridge. That's why if you plan your meals in advance, you will be able to reduce your choices so that you are not tempted to eat anything else. This frees up your mental space so that you can focus on more important things.

Saves you time and energy: People can't seem to follow the ketogenic diet because you do not have the time and energy to cook your meals at home. But if you do meal prepping, you only need a few hours each week to prepare everything. This saves you time and energy on preparing and figuring out what to eat on a daily basis.

Grocery shopping becomes easier: Planning your meals in advance allows you to know which ingredients you need to buy. You can easily make a list of what you need to buy so that you don't buy other food ingredients not needed for that week of meal prepping.

Saves money: Didn't you know that you can save money with meal prepping? Meal prepping allows you to check your inventory and see if there are ingredients in your fridge that you can use. But more than effectively use your inventory, you can also make a lot of savings if you buy items in bulk.

You stay in the state of ketosis effectively: One of the biggest benefits that you can get from the ketogenic diet is that you will be able to stay in ketosis more effectively. To stay in ketosis, you need to keep track of your macros to make sure that you are eating the right proportion of fats, protein, and carbohydrates. The thing is, meal prepping allows you to calculate your macros ahead of time, so you don't need to calculate every time you consume your meals.

Storage containers

These are important for storing the cooked food. Once the meals are cooked, store them separately in air-tight containers preferably those that are microwavable. Storing them in individual containers allow you to serve food by the time that you want to eat them. Moreover, storing them in separate containers means less exposure to contaminants.

Tips to Stick to Vegan Keto Meal Prep

Make simple recipes

Opting for a one-pot dish can save you a lot of time and energy. Don't be too ambitious in the kitchen unless you are confident enough in your kitchen skills.

Determine your goal

Losing weight is the primary reason why you want to do meal prepping. But aside from that, what are your other goals? Do you want to follow a plant-based ketogenic diet or do clean eating? By knowing what your goals are, you can customize your meal prepping plans that will work for you.

Add some scheduling at the start

At the beginning, it's essential to embed bulk cooking into your daily routines. Schedule a couple of hours at the weekend and set a reminder in your calendar to make sure that you don't end up remembering about your plan to start meal prep on a busy Monday morning. It's not that easy at the start, but as you get further and see all the advantages of pre-made meals, this will feel like a delighting possibility rather than a boring chore.

Get a company

A great way not to give up and to make Meal Preps cooking more fun is to get a good company. Haven't you got a friend or two who also would like to make their life more comfortable and healthier? Get them in! Plan, buy and cook the Preps together to enjoy both opportunities of cheaper no-stress meals and time with your friends.

Use a spreadsheet

Planning ahead becomes so much easier if you use the right tool – the spreadsheet. Don't be afraid to be called a nerd or an OCD just because you are so serious about your meal prepping plans. By using a spreadsheet, you will not only be able to make a meal plan but you can also use it to create a shopping list and calculate your macros.

Stock up your kitchen with the right tools

Meal prepping is serious business and you need the right tools to get everything done. If you have a functional kitchen, then you already have the basics – pots, pans, instant pot, slow cooker, knives, ladles, and others. The tools that you need to stock up on are containers to store your food and enough space in the fridge to keep your food for longer.

Know your macros

Knowing your macros is very important when making meal prep recipes. You can use nutrient calculators online.

Mix and match your food

Eating the same meals daily can eventually bore your palate. When doing meal prep recipes, make sure that you cook not only one ingredient but three or four. That way, you can mix and match your food so that you get different flavors every week. So, for instance, if you made roasted chicken, make sure that you steam vegetables as well or make cauliflower rice.

Having passed all the way from Keto Meal Prep newbies not knowing from where to start and to experienced premade food chefs who are looking forward to cooking some delicious meals for the week to come, we have collected some more great tips for you, to make your way even smoother and happier.

Renew your container park

Storing pre-made meals can become a real pain in the neck if you don't have enough convenient containers. Just imagine sticking foods in pans in plates and then trying to get them all in the fridge - isn't that a disaster. Don't make it hard on yourself and do invest in several microwave and dishwasher compatible container sets. This is a one-time investment that will return to you with lots of saved time and space.

Get you multicooker out

Multicooker can really be of huge help when it comes to Keto Meal Prep. Soups, sauces, casseroles and other slow-cooked meals can make a big part of your prep diet. Just toss all the ingredients in the cooker and feel free to do some other thing, watch a film or lie on a sofa enjoying weekend laziness while your food is getting ready. Cool it down and store in the fridge.

Shape your basic menu

As you are making and trying different meals, pay attention to how you feel about each of them. Have you really liked it? Have you got tired of some ingredients by the end of the week? What has been the best meal of the week? Which dish has been a failure? Repeat the best pieces in other week's menus and diversify it adding some new meals. This way, you will not only be sure to find something that you definitely will like but eventually will get some core recipes that you can always rely on. Finally, you will probably even memorize those and will be able to buy necessary ingredients and cook them without any aids.

Arrange theme days

For some of us, making up a menu may be of more burden and effort than actually cooking food. If this is the case, theme days may become an excellent solution for you! For example, make Monday a taco day, Tuesday a sandwich day, Wednesday a fish day, etc. This is not really a must, but it can really make planning your menu easier.

Use overlapping ingredients

Buying in bulk is always cheaper, so consider using the same ingredient for different meals: carrots, onion, tomatoes... even meat can be bought once and used in many dishes. All you need to do is keep in mind the list of ingredients from the previous day when you are planning the next one.

Chapter 5   Benefits of Meal Planning for Beginners

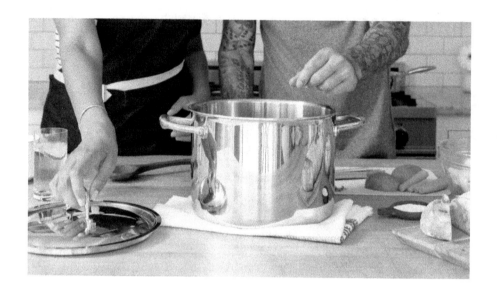

After utilizing the labels on the containers, it becomes apparent that most people need to incorporate a healthy meal plan into their diet. As such, tools are often available not only in print form but also in videos, as well as three-dimensional models that can assist in training, as well as teaching students in becoming more conscious about their health. Therefore, learners seeking to incorporate the appropriate meal planning ideas need to look for a viable option that will help them in supporting their quest to live better lives. Some clients are not in a position to select or even master the right skills for preparing a meal. Such individuals need the assistance of a professional meal planner in incorporating a reliable meal plan. With that said, there are about three meal planning tools that can be used by professionals. No matter how much some people are educated on matters of indulging in a healthy diet, some are often lagging behind when it comes to eating right. Therefore, they seek the usefulness of having a meal planning professional who can assist them in incorporating a new diet plan.

Trained people may find meal planning to be a major barrier to some of their meaningful diet plans. In 1989, the American Association of Diabetics launched the initial Month of Meals manuscript. Some of the books that provided low-fat, as well as low-calorie menus are abundant in many ways. Menus that did not meet the requirements and demands of individuals who lack the necessary skills, as well as interest to prepare meals were included in the book in order to empower such people to seek better menu plans in the long run. As such, it was also discovered that various people in the study catered to their needs by checking out some of the meals that were incorporated in the new healthy menus that seek to improve the health of other people.

According to the cardiovascular risk education and dietary interventions trial, people with diabetes are vastly experiencing tremendous difficulties in getting the right meals to prepare at home. Not only do they seek the help of different professionals but also the input of various people in the sector. In the long run, these individuals are focused on getting help. The professionals in charge of the dietary recommendations are also taking a significant role in helping people to identify different meal planning options that can help in providing solutions for better lives. As such, the trial majorly compared stable versus complex dietary recommendations in various meals. The trial is also at the core of everything when it comes to identifying basic nutritional elements to incorporate in the meal planning charts and graphs. As such, the program was guided toward initiating a proper meal planning session that lasted a significant number of days in a particular homestead. Also, the meal program resulted in relatively more significant weight loss, coupled with the reduction in consumer's blood pressure. This is when compared to the other significant interventions found in the initial trial of the meal planning program.

Based on these findings, it was also discovered that the usual standard of the meal planning programs was observed by many people in the families. The need to offer more specific information to assist people in weight loss that fits perfectly into the objectives of meal planning. For beginners, this is a big deal since the idea seeks to help learners in identifying different meal planning strategies that can support their health in different ways. For this reason, these people can easily seek the assistance of a health professional who is also a guru when it comes to identifying meal planning ideas. Most people recover from concerns related to high blood pressure after indulging in healthier meals. Two more interventions were included in the diet plan to assist the people to watch their weight in different ways that could support their health and well-being. Therefore, their glucose levels were also standardized in many ways.

The need to be more specific when it comes to meal planning and dieting is highly related to seeking health in the long run. The focus on the need to be more specific is also a major move toward providing healthier living standards for the people. Today's nutrition counsellors have also learned how to engage different people in helpful meal planning and encouraging them to develop a variety of skills intended to support their growth, as well as development, especially when it comes to selecting health-based diets. As such, it has become important to teach the fundamentals of cutting down dietary fats in various meals. To participate in the change of eating habits, counseling has become important in the sense that it involves more than a selected education technique and practice in the long run. To this end, a review in the research studies clearly indicated that it is important for learners to adhere to different lessons that would encourage them to adapt to new eating habits. The critical dissemination of this information, as well as training on different meal planning skills, is effective when it comes to changing a person's eating behavior. In new studies, it was also proposed that developing this knowledge is important for the masses. With such knowledge, the current nutritional counselor has to be pretty adept and prepared as much as possible, especially when it comes to identifying some of the basics of catering to different categories of people.

With more reviews being observed from different corners of the world, it has also been discovered that the health basics of different people are a result of the much they consume not only in terms of portions but also the type of meals they take. To change their eating habits, these individuals need the knowledge to select health meals, even from fast-food restaurants. Selected education techniques must also be included in nutritional studies. As such, a review of the same has established that many research studies have not been effective when it comes to changing the eating disorders that affected many people in society. Behavioral change was also discussed as the main agenda when it comes to incorporating new eating habits in different people. Teaching these people to adopt new eating styles is the main agenda for many health professionals who aspire to take up new roles in society by guiding people to eat healthy meals. Only in research studies where different people were successfully preparing and eating healthy meals, as well as diets. To change their eating habits, as well as nutritional focus, these individuals are highly encouraged to seek the attention and guidance of a reliable meal planner who can assist in meal organization. Other than that, it has become vital for such individuals to seek the help of a nutritional service provider who is a professional in the catering department. Only in certain studies where the participants were self-selected and motivated that the people were tasked with the responsibility of finding out if they could engage in behavioral components and therapy, skills, as well as training in order to come up with a reliable eating pattern that mainly focused on health-based diets.

The introduction of these eating patterns marked the onset of healthy eating in many people's lives. Most of the individuals who participated in the research studies played a role in determining a healthy diet, including how they should be developed. The knowledge, behavior, as well as communication models were also used in determining the behavioral components of the subjects. Unfortunately, after the study, it was established that the results provided by the scientific professionals would intensely affect the health of the consumers in various ways. Participants were also tasked with the responsibility of watching what they ate in many ways, including indulging in a diet that would support their weight loss journey. The knowledge, as well as attitude and behavior, were some of the elements that were incorporated in assessing the technique of incorporating meal planning in various programs. As such, it was also discovered in the studies that it was possible for people to indulge in new feeding ideas in many ways. Other than that, different people also delved into the meal planning programs to watch over their health. Meal planning could also be a significant program toward helping people to address the issue of time scarcity. Notably, the method of planning meals for other people is a way toward which others can improve their health by implementing meal preparation in different ways.

It has also been discussed by different meal planners who have taken up the career officially that the idea behind starting different meal feeding programs is geared toward assisting the citizens of different states to incorporate a reliable meal planning program to cater to their families. Apart from that, meal planning can also be used in ensuring that the family is well-fed. As such, the individuals who have implemented meal planning are credited with inventing a new way through which people can engage in healthier diets. Meal planning has continued to receive tremendous attention from different families across different walks of life. There are people who have devoted themselves in ensuring that there is always an appropriate meal planning idea in the process of starting a day. Other families implement meal planning into their lives to help them stay away from lifestyle diseases, such as diabetes and high blood pressure.

According to a survey that was conducted by the health professionals of different universities in the United

States of America, meal planning has become one of the best feeding programs that various families can engage in when seeking to live healthier and better lives. As such, meal planning for beginners has been the talk of different countries across the world. Mothers are joining the program in order to learn more about how to incorporate their meal prepping ideas into a successful meal and dieting plan for the families. Also, the aim of these individuals becoming part of the meal planning programs is for their families to enjoy healthier meals. The cross-sectional studies conducted by different researchers who have been preparing meals for clients and families were conducted to assess people's ability to become part of meal planning programs. It includes adherence to diet and planning, nutritional guidelines, food variety, and weight status. Meal planning has several health benefits.

The first one is learning how to control your portion in different ways. As such, planning your meals will be a way forward in allowing you to have a vision of how you are going to eat. The meal planning idea is going to largely determine how you will indulge in the meal planning process in the long run. In this respect, to become an excellent meal planner, you'll need to consider incorporating the help of a professional in catering for your food. In most cases, the meal planning idea is included to assist you in providing for your meals. You may also be in control of where you will eat because you will be eating at home most of the time. In the long run, regardless of the idea you have in mind based on what you would like to eat, you need to be knowledgeable about meal planning ideas and what it takes to engage in a meal planning program.

Meal planning is also a way toward ensuring that you stay away from fast-food restaurants that may end up serving dishes that can contribute to weight gain in various ways. When an individual is hungry, their blood sugar tremendously drops. Besides that, restaurants are known for serving bigger portions compared to the ones that can be controlled from a home kitchen. With meal planning, you will also be better equipped to cater to your hunger by eating healthy meals and snacks. It is actually one of the best strategies for watching weight. With that said, meal planning is also a significant way through which people can eliminate issues related to weight gain and other health problems that can affect a person. Since people are tied to busy schedules most of the time, including work and school, they may find it challenging to prepare whole foods. This is where meal planning ideas come in to rescue the entire situation. If people can take time to prepare some of these healthy meals, they will be in a position to create a reliable grocery list that can be used by the family. Some of these items are whole grains, beans, as well as fruits and greens. These are not only convenient when it comes to preparation but healthy in all ways possible. As mentioned, meal planning is also a significant time-saver.

In many cases, a busy person will realize that they have nothing planned for dinner. Therefore, it would be useful to have a plan ahead of the actual dinner time instead of waiting until it is time to prepare a meal to eat, especially if it has to be prepared for the family. When it comes to saving money in meal preparation, it is clear that most people can easily economize their money by planning their meals ahead. As such, these people can also engage in several meal planning ideas that can support their nutritional needs. While other people skip meals because of the expenses that come with eating out, meal planning becomes a vital aspect that helps others in preparing for their meals ahead of time. This implies that they shall be in a position to purchase items, such as food ingredients, in bulk. This can also be a great money saver in plenty of ways. Meal planning is also a major tool for getting organized when it comes to shopping for a variety of groceries. Sticking to the list of meals to prepare helps you to pick out what you intend to cook in the long run. You will also be in a position to evade impulse buying. If you are on Instagram, then you have gone through different profiles and observed regular posts on the perfect food preparation and what it takes to prepare the right meals. In the time-lapse videos, you have watched different people implementing different cooking ideas and meal preparation.

However, there is more to food preparation than the actual videos that you observe in the internet. While many people claim to be able to prepare a quick fix for dinner, but it takes more than a whip to come up with a healthy meal for your family. Meal planning involves going to the store and picking items that you are supposed to use in the preparation of dinner and other meals. You should stick to what has been written on the list to reduce the risk of impulse buying. Meal planning is also one of the few strategies that can be used by people who would like to avoid wasting their food. With this idea, you can easily walk into a shop and purchase all the variety of ingredients that you need in your meal preparation process. Avoid food wastage by creating a list of food products that you will need for a week or so.

Whether you intend to cook for the whole family or yourself, taking some time in planning your meals for the week is, of course, one of the most fundamental strategies you can use in meal planning. When it comes to planning for your meals for the week, you should really look into how to get the actual items. Not only will this save you the time needed in planning, but it will also fetch you the right ideas intended for meal planning in the end. When your meals have an intended purpose, you do not need to worry about the items that are stocked in your fridge. You will always be focused in acquiring the right items for your dinner plans. The plan is to create some time and come up with a list for your products. It is also vital for you to go to the store and shop for them by yourself. This is a move toward ensuring that you are getting the right items for your meal preparation.

Chapter 6   Breakfast

Almond Joy Microwave Muffin

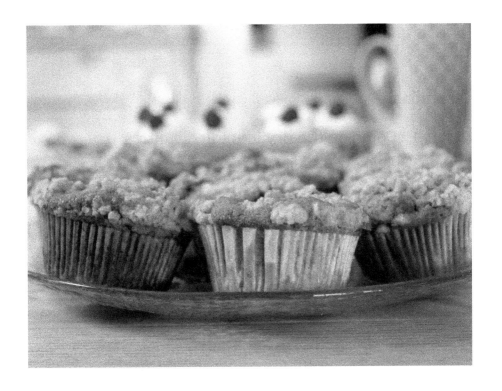

Prep time: 3 min; Cook time: 1 min

Serving Size: 1; Serves: 1; Calories: 207

Total Fat: 16.8g; Protein: 9.7g; Total Carbs: 3.7g

Dietary Fiber: 3; Sugar: 0; Sodium: 300mg

Ingredients

- 2 T almond flour
- 1 tsp Coconut Flour

- 1 packet Splenda
- 1/4 tsp Baking Powder
- Sprinkle of Salt
- 1 Egg
- 1 T butter
- 1 tsp cocoa

Directions

1. Combine the dry ingredients into a microwaveable mug.
2. Quickly whip the egg and the oil together.
3. Stir into the dry mixture.
4. Microwave on high for 1 minute.
5. Toast with butter.

Prep Instructions

Place all dry ingredients in zip-lock baggies, 1 recipe per bag. Do not premix the eggs and oil. Wait until morning for combining.

Black and Blue Smoothie

Prep time: 4 min; Cook time: 0 min

Serving Size: 1; Serves: 1; Calories: 221

Total Fat: 9.8g; Protein: 21.8g; Total Carbs: 10g

Dietary Fiber: 5.8g; Sugar: 1g; Sodium: 0mg

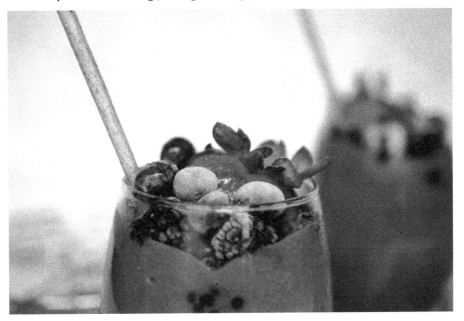

Ingredients

- ¼ cup Frozen Blueberries
- ¼ cup Frozen Blackberries
- 1 C unsweetened soy or almond milk
- 1 tsp vanilla
- 1 scoop (your choice) vanilla whey protein powder
- 2 packets sweetener of your choice

- 3 tsp flaxseeds

Directions

1. Mix the ingredients and emulsify by blending.
2. Pulse four times or until desired thickness.
3. Pour into a glass and enjoy.

Prep Instructions

Combine berries in freezer bags and place in the freezer. Combine sweetener of your choice, flaxseeds, and protein powder in zip-lock bags. Combine milk and vanilla in 1 cup containers in the fridge.

Breakfast Casserole

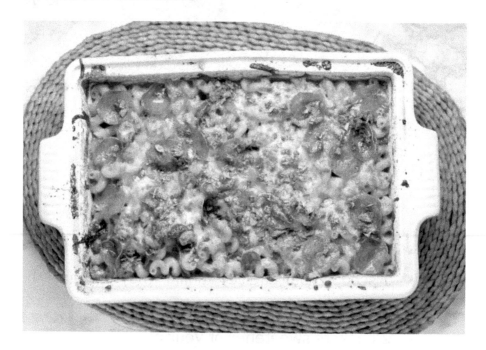

Prep time: 4 min; Cook time: 19 min

Serving Size: 1 dish; Serves: 4; Calories: 195

Total Fat: 11g; Protein: 19g; Total Carbs: 3g

Dietary Fiber: 1g; Sugar: 0; Sodium: 112mg

Ingredients

- 8 oz Sausage, Cooked and Crumbled
- 1 cup hot salsa
- 4 eggs
- 2 chopped green onions
- ¼ cup hand-shredded pepper jack or cheddar cheese
- ½ bell pepper, chopped, your choice of color

Directions

1. Place oven rack to the middle shelf setting.
2. Heat oven to 400 degrees.
3. Cook the peppers until soft.
4. Spray or grease the baking dishes excessively. Eggs stick when baked.
5. Layer ingredients in 4 individual baking dishes, like Corning ware "grab-its", any bakeware that holds one cup servings.
6. Layer with sausage first, then peppers, then cheese.

7. Add one whipped egg to each baking dish.
   Sprinkle with green onions.

8. Bake for 18 minutes, until eggs are set.

Freezing Instructions

Place cooled casseroles in individual freezer bags.
Reheat in microwave for 2-3 minutes until hot.

Breakfast Mexican Omelet

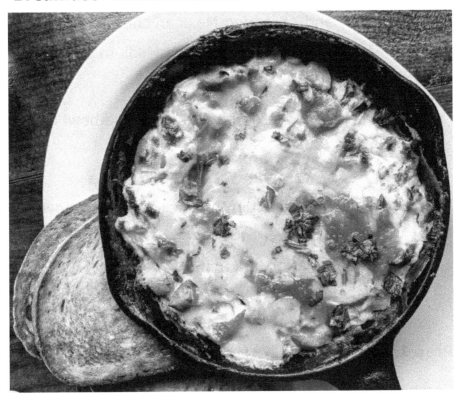

Prep time: 4 min; Cook time: 9 min

Serving Size: 1; Serves: 1; Calories: 275

Total Fat: 21; Protein: 17g; Total Carbs: 3.2g

Dietary Fiber: 2g; Sugar: 2g; Sodium: 230mg

Ingredients

- ½ T lime juice
- 2 eggs
- 1 tsp water
- 1 T crumbled bacon

- 1/2 T butter
- ¼ avocado
- ½ c hand-shredded Mexican cheese
- 2 T Pace Thick and Chunky Medium Salsa

Directions

1. Melt the butter in a microwaveable bowl in the microwave.
2. Quickly whip the wet ingredients in a microwaveable bowl, can be the same bowl as before.
3. Microwave for one minute.
4. Place on warm plate.
5. Top with all the rest of the ingredients.

Prep Instructions

Combine the wet ingredients in a zip-lock bag, except the butter and water. Refrigerate. Combine the water and butter in a zip-lock bag.

Butter Pecan Waffles

Prep time: 9 min; Cook time: 4 min

Serving Size: 1; Serves: 8; Calories: 181

Total Fat: 13g; Protein: 9g; Total Carbs: 5g

Dietary Fiber: 2g; Sugar: 3g; Sodium: 178mg

Ingredients

- 1 cup soy flour
- 2 packets Splenda
- 3 tsp baking powder
- ¾ cup buttermilk
- 1 T butter
- ½ tsp baking soda
- 3 eggs
- 2 T vanilla
- ½ cup water
- 2 T sugar free butter rum flavoring
- ½ c pecans

Directions

1. Combine everything except the pecans.
2. Use ¼ c batter for cooking the waffle.
3. Cook until crisp.
4. Top with pecans and sugar free syrup.

Freezing Instructions

After the waffle is cool, place 1 per zip-lock bag. Warm by toasting in the toaster.

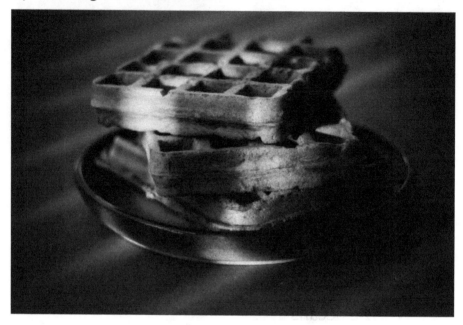

Chapter 7   Lunch

Albacore Tuna Vinaigrette Salad

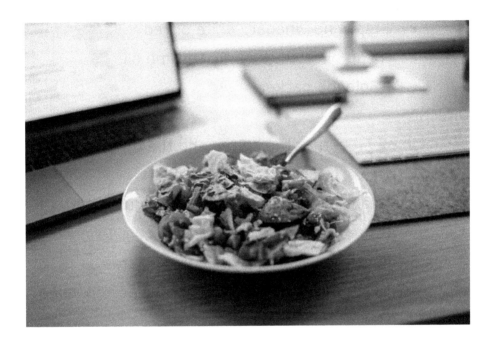

Prep time: 10 min; Cook time: 7 min

Serving Size: 1/4; Serves: 4; Calories: 231

Total Fat: 20g; Protein: 9g; Total Carbs: 5.5g

Dietary Fiber: 5g; Sugar: 0g; Sodium: 265mg

Ingredients

- 1 can albacore tuna, drained
- 1 pound of fresh or frozen asparagus
- ¼ cup walnuts, chopped
- 4 cups baby salad mix
- ½ tsp salt

- ¼ tsp pepper
- 3 tsp finely chopped onion
- 1 tsp spicy brown mustard
- 2 tsp wine vinegar, white or red
- ¼ cup olive oil or garlic sesame oil
- 1 Splenda packet

Directions

1. Mix together the spices and the tuna, set aside.
2. Steam the asparagus for 5-7 minutes until desired crispness.
3. Place the salad mixture onto 4 plates.
4. Divide the asparagus by 4 and place on salad greens.
5. Divide the seasoned tuna by 4 and scatter onto the asparagus and salad.
6. Sprinkle each salad with the walnuts and serve.

Prep Instructions

Place the tuna mixture in a zip-lock bag and place in the fridge. Steam the asparagus and place in a zip-lock bag in the fridge. Place the salad mix in zip-locks in the fridge. Put the walnuts in a bag in the fridge.

Barbecue Chicken Pizza

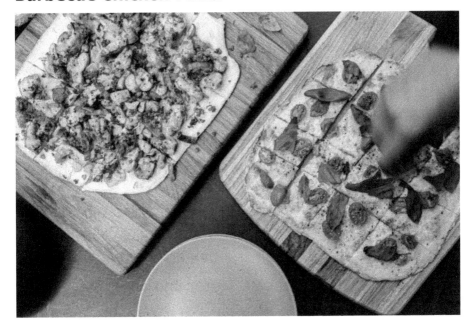

Prep time: 19 min; Cook time: 29 min

Serving Size: 1 pizza; Serves: 8 Calories: 285

Total Fat: 12g; Protein: 27g Total Carbs: 7g

Dietary Fiber: 5g; Sugar: 0g; Sodium: 100mg

Ingredients

- 1/2 cup G Hughes Smokehouse BBQ Sauce, sugar free
- ½ tsp salt
- 2 cups baking mix, low-carb
- 1 cup water
- 1 chopped red onion
- 1 cup cooked chicken, diced

- ½ cup chopped bell peppers, red, green, yellow assortment
- ½ cup sliced black olives
- 3 T olive oil
- 1 cup mozzarella cheese, hand-shredded
- ½ c parmesan cheese, hand-shredded
- 1 packet Splenda or sweetener of your choice

Directions

1. Set oven to 425 F.
2. Mix into a dough the baking powder, baking mix, Splenda, salt, water and oil.
3. Place on waxed paper and lightly oil. Roll into your pizza crust.
4. Bake for 9 minutes.
5. Remove from heat source and spread the barbecue sauce onto the crust.
6. Layer the toppings, placing the cheeses on top.
7. Bake 15 more minutes until thoroughly warmed and the cheese is melted.
8. Slice into 8 pieces and serve.

Freezing Directions

Place individual slices in a zip-lock freezer bag. Freeze. To serve, heat in microwave one minute.

Chicken Lettuce Wraps

Prep time: 10min; Cook time: 10min

Serving Size: 1; Serves: 1; Calories: 145

Total Fat: 1g; Protein: 35g; Total Carbs: 4g

Dietary Fiber: 1g; Sugar: 0g; Sodium: 100mg

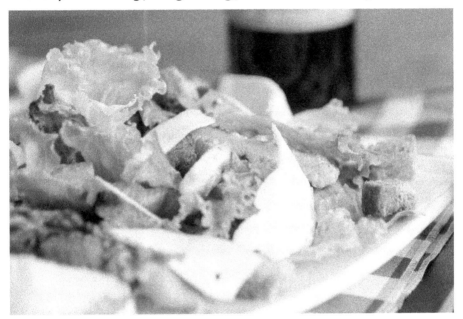

Ingredients

- 1 chicken breast, boneless, diced into 1-inch size pieces
- 1 cup diced or sliced fresh mushrooms
- ½ cup diced water chestnuts (from a can, drained)
- 1 T olive oil

- 1 T onion, minced
- 1 T minced garlic
- 1 T teriyaki sauce
- garlic powder, only a dash
- onion powder, just a dash
- oregano, one dash
- cayenne pepper, a small dash
- salt /pepper

Directions

1. Mix the ingredients and cook in a skillet until the chicken is done, about 10 minutes.
2. Shred the chicken
3. Place in leaves and roll

Freezing Instructions

Place all ingredients into one freezer bag except the lettuce. Microwave one minute and serve.

Chicken Quesadillas

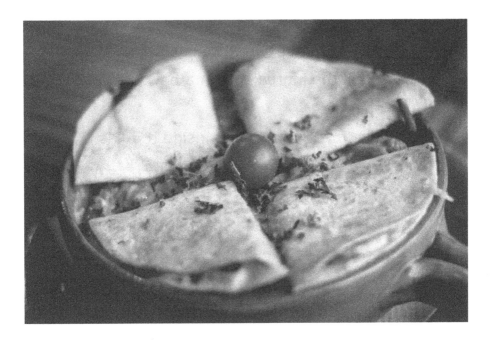

Prep time: 4 min; Cook time: 4 min

Serving Size: 1; Serves: 4; Calories: 425g

Total Fat: 25g; Protein: 44g; Total Carbs: 10g

Dietary Fiber: 9g; Sugar: 2g; Sodium: 186mg

Ingredients

- 1 cup pepper jack cheese, hand-shredded
- 8 tortillas Tortilla Factory Low Carb Whole Wheat Tortillas
- 8 oz. cooked and shredded Chicken Breast
- 1 chopped and Roasted Bell Pepper
- 2 T Cilantro

- 2 T Butter
- 1 cup plain Greek yogurt

Directions

1. Place ½ pat of butter in a skillet
2. Mix all the ingredients in a bowl except the yogurt
3. Place meat ingredients inside tortillas
4. Toast each side
5. Cut into 4 wedges
6. Top with yogurt and salsa, if desired

Freezing Instructions

Freeze in zip-lock bags. Place the yogurt in the fridge. Heat one minute in microwave to thaw.

Chili Mac

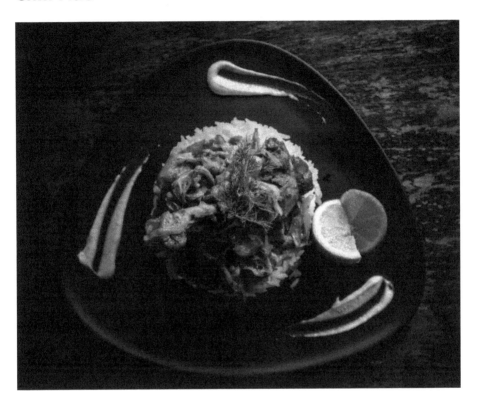

Prep time: 9 min; Cook time: 9 min

Serving Size: 1/4; Serves: 4; Calories: 480

Total Fat: 24g; Protein: 36g; Total Carbs: 25g

Dietary Fiber: 6g; Sugar: 4g; Sodium: 995mg

Ingredients

- 1 lb ground Sirloin
- 1 chopped Onion
- 1 Chili Seasoning Mix, packet

- 1 cup tomato sauce
- 1 small can of Chunky Diced Tomatoes & Green Chilies
- 1 cup hand-shredded sharp cheddar
- 1 packet Splenda
- ½ cup Barilla Proteinplus Elbow macaroni

Directions

1. Boil Barilla Proteinplus Elbow macaroni until done, drain.
2. Brown the sirloin and onions in a large skillet.
3. Add the pasta, tomato sauce, diced tomatoes and green chilies, and chili seasoning mix.
4. Taste to see if you need to add water.
5. Serve in 4 bowls, topping each bowl with the cheddar cheese.

Freezer Directions

Place in four containers with lids, freeze. Microwave 2 minutes to thaw.

Cream of Mushroom Soup

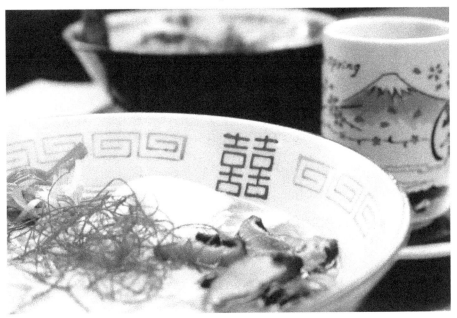

Prep time: 6 min; Cook time: 4 min
Serving Size: 1 cup; Serves: 4; Calories: 210

Total Fat: 17g; Protein: 10g; Total Carbs: 3g

Dietary Fiber: 0.5g; Sugar: 0g; Sodium: 370mg

Ingredients

- 1 pound mushrooms, sliced
- 1 T butter
- ¼ cup cream
- 1 cup water
- ¼ grated Parmesan cheese
- dash of basil
- dash of black pepper

Directions

1. Microwave the mushrooms in the water for 4 minutes. Taste for desired doneness.
2. Drain the mushrooms.
3. Place in blender with butter and cream and Parmesan.
4. Blend until creamy.
5. Pour into bowl and serve

Freezing Instructions

Freeze cooked soup in one cup containers. Microwave one minute, stir, and microwave one more minute to serve.

Chapter 8   Dinner

Beef Stroganoff with Protein Noodles

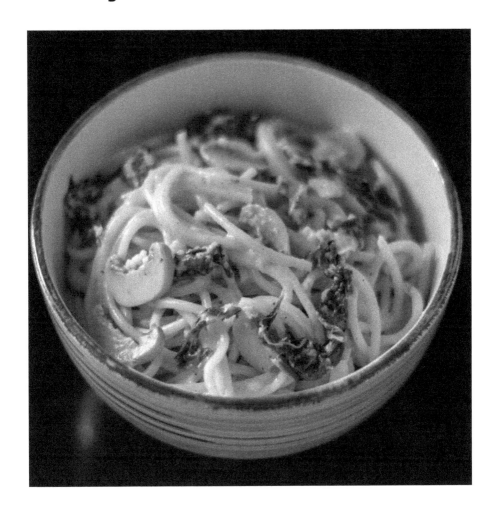

Prep time: 14 min; Cook time: 29 min

Serving Size: 1; Serves: 1; Calories: 559

Total Fat: 23g; Protein: 55g; Total Carbs: 4g

Dietary Fiber: 13g; Sugar: 2g; Sodium: 957mg

Ingredients

- 2 oz. Barilla Protein Farfalle Pasta
- ½ cup fresh sliced mushrooms
- 2 Tbls of chopped onion
- 1 T butter
- dash of black pepper
- 6 oz. steak, sliced thinly
- 1 T tomato paste
- ¼ tsp of Dijon mustard
- ½ cup beef broth
- ½ small container plain Greek yogurt

Directions

1. Cook the pasta in water.
2. Place the butter in a Teflon skillet.
3. Next add in the onions, and mushrooms, cook until onions are shiny and water is gone.
4. Add the beef and brown well.
5. Stir in remaining ingredients except the pasta and yogurt.
6. Cook this until the beef is done, approximately 9 minutes.
7. Drain the pasta.
8. If the sauce is too thin, add 1 tsp low carb flax meal and boil to thicken.

9. Turn back down to low. Then add the yogurt to the sauce.

10. Serve the stroganoff over the pasta.

Freezing Instructions

Place dish in appropriate container with a lid and freeze. Heat 2 minutes in a microwave to serve.

Beefy Tostadas

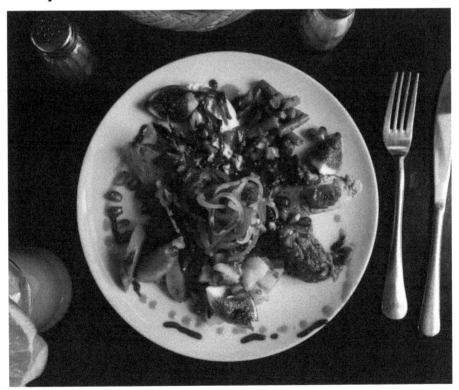

Prep time: 4 min; Cook time: 9 min

Serving Size: 2 tostadas; Serves: 1; Calories: 735

Total Fat: 48g; Protein: 66g; Total Carbs: 18g

Dietary Fiber: 8g; Sugar: 0g; Sodium: 708mg

Ingredients

- ¼ pound ground sirloin
- ¼ cup onions, minced
- 1 tsp garlic, minced
- 1 T olive oil
- ½ cup chopped green, red, and yellow peppers
- ½ cup cheddar cheese, mild or sharp, hand-shredded
- 2 Tortilla factory low-carb tortillas
- 2 T butter
- 1 c Greek yogurt, plain
- 2 T salsa verde

Directions

1. Brown the tortillas in the butter. Place on a warm plate.
2. Cook the sirloin, onions, garlic, peppers in the olive oil.
3. Place on the tortillas.
4. Top with the cheese.
5. Add the Greek yogurt.
6. Drizzle with the salsa.

Freezing Directions

Freeze the serving of the meat mixture in a zip-lock bag. Microwave on a plate for one minute to serve. Place the cheese in a zip-lock bag. Add the salsa and the yogurt if you desire. Place the tortillas between wet paper towels and microwave the refrigerated tortillas for 15 seconds before serving.

Bratwurst German Dinner

Prep time: 4 min; Cook time: 19 min

Serving Size: 1; Serves: 1; Calories: 332

Total Fat: 26g; Protein: 15g; Total Carbs: 8g

Dietary Fiber: 9g; Sugar: 4g; Sodium: 1188mg

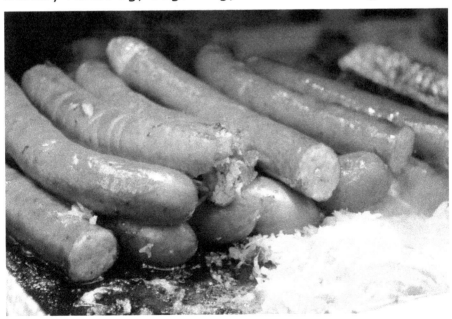

Ingredients

- 1 Bratwurst sausage
- ½ cup sliced onion
- ½ cup sauerkraut, this includes the liquid
- 1 tsp olive oil
- Sprinkle of black pepper

Directions

1. Cook the bratwurst and the onion in the olive oil, in a coated skillet.
2. Remove the bratwurst to a plate.
3. Place the sauerkraut into the skillet and cook 3 min.
4. Add the bratwurst and onion back to warm and mingle the flavors.
5. Sprinkle with black pepper and serve.

Freezing Directions

Place entire serving in one freezer zip-lock bag. Reheat in microwave for 2 minutes.

Cajun Blackened Fish with Cauliflower Salad

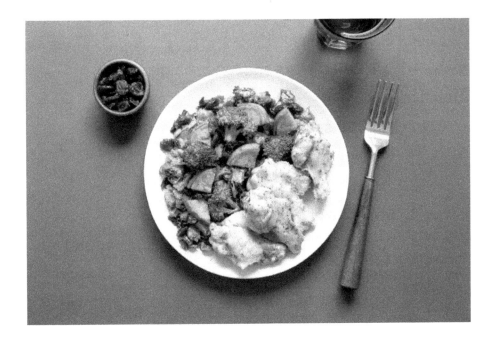

Prep time: 9 min; Cook time: 9 min

Serving Size: 1; Serves: 1; Calories: 530

Total Fat: 33.5g; Protein: 32g; Total Carbs: 5.5g

Dietary Fiber: 4g; Sugar: 3g; Sodium: 80mg

Ingredients

- 1 cup chopped cauliflower
- 1 tsp red pepper flakes
- 1 T Italian seasonings
- 1 T garlic, minced
- 6 oz. tilapia
- 1 cup English cucumber, chopped with peel
- 2 T olive oil

- 1 sprig dill, chopped
- 1 Sweetener packet
- 3 T lime juice
- 2 T Cajun blackened seasoning

Directions

1. Mix the seasonings, except the Cajun blackened seasoning, into one bowl.
2. Add 1 T olive oil.
3. Emulsify or whip.
4. Pour the dressing over the cauliflower and cucumber.
5. Brush the fish with the olive oil on both sides.
6. Pour the other 1 T oil into a coated skillet.
7. Press the Cajun seasoning onto both sides of the fish.
8. Cook the fish in the olive oil 3 minutes per side.
9. Plate and serve.

Prep Instructions

Place all the veggies and dressing into one zip-lock bag. Refrigerate.

Freeze each piece of fish individually in a zip-lock bag.

Microwave 30 seconds to serve.

Chicken Parmesan over Protein Pasta

Prep time: 9 min; Cook time: 14 min

Serving Size: 2 oz. pasta, 1 cutlet; Serves: 4; Calories: 372

Total Fat: 18g; Protein: 56g; Total Carbs:7 g

Dietary Fiber: 2g; Sugar: 6g; Sodium: 1335mg

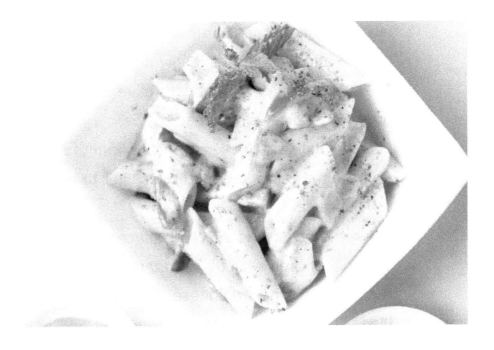

Ingredients

- 1 dash black pepper
- ½ tsp Italian spice mix
- 8 oz. Protein Plus Spaghetti
- ½ hand-shredded Parmesan

- 1 diced zucchini squash
- 1 ½ cups marinara sauce, any brand
- 24 oz. boneless thin chicken cutlets
- 2 T olive oil
- ½ cup grated Mozzarella cheese
- Water, for boiling the pasta

Directions

1. Boil the pasta with the zucchini in the water.
2. Mix the Italian spices and ¼ cup Parmesan cheese and place in a shallow dish.
3. Brush the chicken pieces with olive oil and press into spice and cheese to coat.
4. Place in skillet with the oil and cook until done.
5. Add the marinara sauce to the skillet to warm, cover the chicken if you desire.
6. Drain the pasta and zucchini, place on plates.
7. Top the chicken with the mozzarella and remaining Parmesan cheese.
8. Place sauce, chicken, and cheese onto spaghetti and serve.

Freezing Instructions

Make sure the spaghetti is covered with sauce, then freeze in containers. Microwave 3 minutes to serve.

Chicken Chow Mein Stir Fry

Prep time: 9 min; Cook time: 14 min;

Serving Size: 1/4; Serves: 4; Calories: 368

Total Fat: 18g; Protein: 42g; Total Carbs: 12g

Dietary Fiber: 16g; Sugar: 6g; Sodium: 746mg

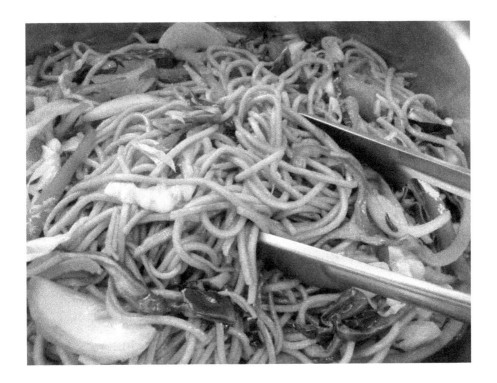

Ingredients

- 1/2 cup sliced onion
- 2 T Oil, sesame garlic flavored
- 4 cups shredded Bok-Choy
- 1 c Sugar Snap Peas

- 1 cup fresh bean sprouts
- 3 stalks Celery, chopped
- 1 1/2 tsp minced Garlic
- 1 packet Splenda
- 1 cup Broth, chicken
- 2 T Soy Sauce
- 1 T ginger, freshly minced
- 1 tsp cornstarch
- 4 boneless Chicken Breasts, cooked/sliced thinly

Directions

1. Place the bok-choy, peas, celery in a skillet with 1 T garlic oil.
2. Stir fry until bok-choy is softened to liking.
3. Add remaining ingredients except the cornstarch.
4. If too thin, stir cornstarch into ½ cup cold water. When smooth pour into skillet.
5. Bring cornstarch and chow mein to a one-minute boil. Turn off the heat source.
6. Stir sauce then for wait 4 minutes to serve, after the chow mein has thickened.

Freezing Directions

Freeze in covered containers. Heat for 2 minutes in the microwave before serving

Colorful Chicken Casserole

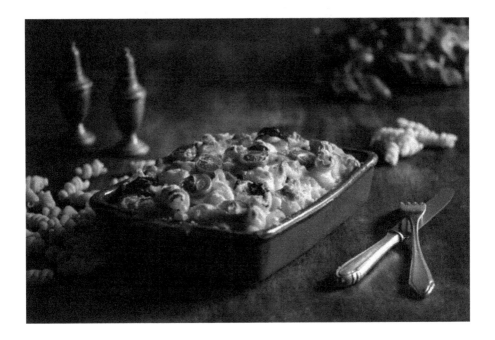

Prep time: 14 min; Cook time: 14 min

Serving Size: 1 cup; Serves: 6; Calories: 412

Total Fat: 30g; Protein: 29; Total Carbs: 10g

Dietary Fiber: 9g; Sugar: 1g; Sodium: 712mg

Ingredients

- 1 cup broth, chicken
- 3 cups cooked chicken, diced
- 4 cups chopped broccoli
- 1 cup assorted colored bell peppers, chopped
- 1 cup cream
- 4 T sherry
- ¼ c hand-shredded Parmesan cheese

- 1 small size can black olives, sliced, drained
- 2 Tortilla Factory low-carb whole wheat tortillas
- ½ c hand-shredded mozzarella

Directions

1. Place broccoli and chicken broth into a skillet.
2. Top with lid, bring to a boil, and steam until desired crispness. (4 min)
3. Add the peppers, steam for one minute if you don't want them crisp.
4. Add the chicken and stir to heat.
5. Combine the sherry, cream, parmesan, and olives.
6. Tear the tortillas into bite-sized pieces.
7. Stir into the chicken and broccoli.
8. Pour cream sauce over the chicken, stir.
9. Top with hand-shredded mozzarella.
10. Broil in oven until cheese is melted and golden brown.

Freezing Directions

Place in covered containers to freeze. Microwave 2 minutes to serve.

Chapter 9   Mindful Eating

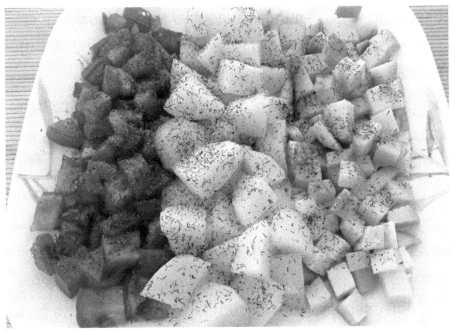

Clean eating basically involves consuming foods that are fresh and natural by way of avoiding processed foods and additives. Clean eating is essential in the sense that, if done effectively, it can boost immunity and one's health in general. Adopting clean eating habits can be achieved by preparing home-cooked meals, which are healthier and have fewer additives. It also allows you to save money.

As reiterated in the chapters, mindful eating is a vital element to consider in your daily routine of food consumption. Mindfulness is a term applied to a person's eating habits. Therefore, mindful eating is the manner in which an individual uses the various acts of mindfulness to overcome issues appended to health. In the long run, the idea is to assist a person to incorporate viable eating methods with the plan to help the consumers of a family to partake in slightly healthier eating routines. Mindful eating is supposed to help a person learn how to consume small to moderate amounts of different macronutrients. Therefore, for one to be successful in eating, they need to be in a position to take what is considered to be healthy.

The objective, in the long run, is to help in shifting focus from the external thinking regarding food to exploring the existing eating experience and settling for a meal plan that can help you to acquire a healthy regimen that can support health. Mindful eating is also considered to be a viable method of assisting you in considering healthier diets. The objective of the plan, in the end, is to assist different people to indulge in better and supportive healthcare systems that can help them consume better meals that can support their well-being. Mindful eating is really a diet-focused orientation that is developed using a new mindset. It is the way in which people decide to focus on watching what they eat regardless of what they are craving. As such, mindful eating can also help in supporting the well-being of different people who have ill health and need to invest in their well-being. At the end of it all, mindful eating is also one of the major ways through which an individual can decide to settle for a better and way viable eating plan.

By definition, mindful eating is a strategy that assists a person to take up different roles in the community and assist people who aspire to indulge in a unique eating experience. This is by using all the existing senses, such as smell, touch, as well as taste. To be safe from the issues that may be developed from reckless eating, most people choose to rely on different eating plans in order to develop muscle and lose excess weight. With mindful eating, the idea is to always focus on witnessing the person's emotional, as well as physical response in terms of food consumption.

This implies that food has a significant impact on a person's health and well-being. Therefore, one needs to consider taking up a new feeding style that suits their reaction to food. This should be considered during and after consuming the meals. With mindful eating, people often watch their weight. They also focus on indulging in various foods that support their health, as well as well-being. Therefore, it is a move toward ensuring that an individual focuses on partaking the right meals every way possible. In the long run, what most people really need to understand is the fact that, with mindful eating, you actually need to observe even the calorie intake and indulge in better calorie quantity.

While at it, it is also important to note that mindful eating may seem like a challenge. As usual, you could be ravenously hungry to hold back the feeling of wanting to feel satiated in the long run. However, with mindful eating, you can largely benefit the body as well as the mind, thereby allowing it to have sufficient time in order to be able to register its ability to be full.

With mindful eating, you shall also realize that it is slightly easy to be able to take on different meals, depending on how beneficial they are to the body. In the long run, you will be able to comprehend the benefits of taking your health seriously. Your body will respond to the goodness of your meals and their macronutrients. As such, your body will also register a relatively required nutrient intake. In the world that is fast-paced, with the technology that is quickly taking over the business sector, it has become important for people to indulge in mindful eating because we are constantly slammed by the busy schedules that may not allow us to partake healthy meals.

People are running a lot of errands to the extent of being incapable of taking in healthy meals in the required amounts. Others are even stuck wondering if they can indulge in healthy diets, given that they have busy schedules. Are these people in a position to get enough nutrients, carbohydrates, as well as vitamins? At the end of it all, it becomes necessary for people to stay happy, as well as healthy. One of the easiest ways to accomplish this is by taking care of one's health and watching what they eat. In the long run, you really want to understand what it takes to be part of healthy meal planning.

Mindful eating is the main way through which you can become sensitive to what you are consuming. To most people, giving the brain sufficient oxygen is a vital element to consider. Therefore, it only becomes possible if mindful eating is considered in the long run. This implies that it is important for people to consider taking the initiative to eat healthily. Apart from that, the family needs to be included in the meal plan of mindful and careful eating.

All this is going to be one of the most important strategies of considerations when it comes to taking the right meal at the right time. With mindful eating, people have been in a position to evade overconsumption.

Since they may eat for different reasons, it means that they often eat even when it is not time to consume any form of meal. Therefore, it also implies that it is necessary for people to indulge in healthy eating. With that said, it is vital to actually consider eating healthy. Instead of just reaching for that snack at any point in time, it is essential to consider taking the right move by implementing the right eating habits.

After learning about the importance of meal planning, it is also good to look into the benefits of meal planning.

The Benefits of Meal Planning

Meal planning comes in handy when a person wants to lose weight to just improve their diet. As long as you are able to follow up on your goals, you will easily gain from the meal planning process. There are many advantages that accrue from meal planning, and some of them include improving your health.

In life, you must plan, or else you will not achieve your goals. When you plan your meals and snacks initially, you will have a higher chance of succeeding. Also, you will have a healthier food choice. Some of the benefits of meal planning are as follows.

1. Learning about Portion Control

When a person plans their own meals, they can keep track of how much they are actually eating. Also, it will be possible to avoid foods from restaurants since they are not part of the meal plan. Some of the restaurants may be serving large portions, and you may deviate from your original meal plan.

2. Eating Healthy

When a person is hungry, their blood sugar drops. They will also be more inclined to eat any type of food that is readily available. In most cases, people may opt for foods from fast-food joints, and the main issue is that they are unhealthy.

Meal planning ensures that people can consume healthy meals. The diet present in a meal plan should also be balanced. It is good to note that, in most instances, people choose unhealthy meals since they are convenient. When people take some time to plan their meals, they can come up with a grocery list that contains vegetables, fruits, whole grains, fruits, and other types of food. It will become more convenient, and a person can lead a healthy lifestyle.

3. Saving Time

When a person is hungry, and they do not have a meal plan or any ready food, they may be stressed. In such an instance, people look for the most convenient type of food that is readily available. When a meal plan is available, it is possible to have a healthy meal ready in minutes. Additionally, ready meals that have been refrigerated ensure that people can save on time, especially when cleaning dishes after cooking.

Ways to Start Eating Clean

Have you always wanted to start eating, but you do not know where to begin? Well, here are some of the ways you can start eating clean.

- Understand why you are eating clean and what value that adds to your life.
- Have a meal plan, which incorporates locally available fresh foods and vegetables. Meal plans help in balancing diet and the right quantity serving.
- Avoid processed food, and if you can't, limit your intake. During processing, they naturally lose their natural state. They have gained added sugar and chemicals which may increase one's chance of getting a heart disease.

- Check labels on packaged foodstuffs to ensure there are no added sugars, chemical preservatives, and fats that are not healthy
- Avoid overconsuming refined carbohydrates, but eat more whole grain foods since they have more fiber and nutrients, thus reducing or rather eliminating inflammation.

Clean Eating Basics

Clean eating is easier said than done, but it can be done if you know how to do it. It basically means that you eat foods that make your body happy, thus making your body able to repair worn out tissues and reduce inflammation. Clean eating starts from the mindset; have a positive attitude and realize that you are doing it for you so that you can have a good health and healthier lifestyle. It is also essential to discuss your clean eating with your doctor before you embrace a clean eating lifestyle.

I will highlight five key clean eating basics here:

☐   Embrace real food. This basically involves purchasing food that is natural and in season. For instance, buy the fruits that are in season, and make your own fresh juice. The same applies to vegetables and whole grains.

☐ Eliminate unhealthy fats. These are also called saturated fats, mostly found in processed and canned foods from dairy, fatty meat, palm oil, and butter. You can start by reducing the intake, then eliminating it from your diet gradually.

☐ Prepare home-cooked meals. This is not only cheaper and can save you money, but it is also more healthy, convenient, and practical. Cooking at home means you can add the right amount of sugar, measure the ingredients, and decide on the right quantity of each serving. It reduces the fear of uncertainty, such as asking yourself: what if they added more? Is it fresh? Home-cooked meal plans can be done daily, weekly, or bi-monthly, depending on your schedule.

☐ Keep yourself hydrated. By this, I don't mean drinking juice or coffee when thirsty but drink lots of water. Most fruits have water, but the body still needs lots and lots of water for healthy digestion, thus avoiding constipation. Being hydrated also boosts heart function. Limit the intake of coffee and alcohol since too much intake of these two beverage types can pose serious health risks, such as anxiety, insomnia, jitteriness, and, in some cases, even stomach upsets.

13 Tips for Clean Eating and Weight Loss

It has been proven that clean healthy not only generates a healthy body but also promotes healthy and productive lifestyle. It can slow down some elements of lifestyle diseases and is also remedy for worn out tissue repair. Clean eating can also be used as weight loss remedy besides exercises. It means you love your body so much, and you are willing to sacrifice and give it what is good for it and what can help it function well without listening to what your taste buds want.

It is clear to note that your mind should be the first to embrace clean eating because your mind will influence your attitude toward the healthy food you will be consuming. Healthy mindset will translate to healthy lifestyle, thus giving you a healthy body and soul. Healthy eating should not mean including an exercise regime in your daily life, but it should be done with exercise, too. That is because exercise also helps tone down the muscles, helps in heartbeat, and removes some salt from the body.

Here are 13 tips for clean eating and weight loss and saving time for your lifestyle, so you can love and heal your body.

1. Be the chief chef

Unleash that inner chef in you. Prepare your whole grain and fresh foods from home, this will help you measure the right quantity needed and also help you avoid the temptation to indulge by eating out. Depending on your schedule, you can even pack your own food if you are working. Fresh foods and vegetable prepared from home are more healthy, nutritious and affordable.

Use locally available foods and stock your refrigerator with the healthy vegetables. Use herbs for seasoning instead of canned seasonings. Finally, enjoy and appreciate your home cooked meal. Be creative, and don't do the same meal every day, check on the nutritional value and serve the right potions.

2. Think green go green

Arugula, kale, and spinach are some of green leafy vegetables that can be served with almost every meal. Their green natural state means they have essential minerals and vitamins and also contain antioxidants, which are necessary for a healthy body. Increase the intake of these because they can also help in detoxification, as well as acting as mineral supplements.

3. Have a meal preparation schedule

You can prepare bulk meal for the week when you have time; this will keep you disciplined, and it can help limit the temptation to dash into a fast-food place for take away since you will know you have cooked food waiting for you. The schedule also help you cook at you convenience and reduce the daily cooking stress.

4. Ingredients are more Important than calories
Some food have high calorie while others are low. One should eat more food that nourish their body rather than stop hunger. Energy-dense food cannot be easily digested; they stay longer in the stomach; thus, they may lead to weight gain. Avocado and nuts, for instance, have a lot of calories but contain useful fats. This means that if you eat them between meals, they keep you satisfied. This is also another way of helping one lose weight the healthy way.

5. Increase protein intake
There are so many reasons that you need to increase protein intake in your diet. High protein diet has been shown to increase metabolism, suppresses hunger, and increase body mass. Most protein meals can be added during any serving, proteins like eggs, fish, poultry, dairy, beans and nuts.

6. Don't be scared to experiment

Adopting clean eating may mean incorporating foods that you were not consuming before. Do not be scared to try out that new recipe; buy those healthy grains or greens that you heard or read about and make them a part of your diet. You never know; it can help you discover your new favorite dish.

7. Make it colorful

We all like rainbow; the combination of the colors makes it beautiful. Healthy food does not have to be ugly and unattractive; you can always make the presentation of your food attractive and appetizing. This can especially be done with salads, berries, red pepper, sweet potato, and turmeric. They are not just colorful, but they also contain essential compounds.

8. Stock your refrigerator and pantry

Organize a week to do grocery shopping and ensure your pantry has enough stock to last you even for a week; this will reduce unnecessary grocery shopping and impulse buying, thus saving you some time. Frozen vegetables and some canned healthy grains can be stored in the freezer so that they do not lose their minerals and nutrients.

9. Intuitive eating habit

This basically involves listening to your body and responding to hunger, as well as satisfaction, which, in turn, promotes healthy eating and reduce the chances of overeating, thus boosting mental health as well.

This means you eat when you need to and not just when you have to. Intuitive eating also helps in weight loss, as it prevents unnecessary eating.

10.   Buy organic and local products

Going organic does not only help in saving planet, but organic foods are also very healthy and free from harmful chemicals. Going organic also assist in promoting biodiversity and will help you get information as to which products have harmful pesticides and herbicides.

11.   Liaise with local farmers

There is no better place to get fresh produce than from local farms. Identify farmers nearby and purchase directly from them; you will not only be guaranteed fresh produce but also good pricing. Fresh produce consumed directly from the farm means getting the most of the nutrients; it also means you support and appreciate your local economy.

12.   Eat healthy when you eat out

When you eat out or buy take away, make sure you also order for healthy foods. For instance, swap that ice cream for fruit salad; let your meal have vegetables, too. Avoid fatty foods and high-carbohydrate food in your order.

13.   Set goals, and stick to them

Clean eating requires a lot of discipline, hard work, and focus. Once you begin, do not look back, and stick to your meal plan. Network with friends or join groups of people eating healthy to get that moral support. And every week, if you managed to achieve your goal, reward yourself. Also, let people you stay with (if do not live alone) know that you want to eat healthy; they may have the same interest and even do it with you.

These 13 tips are just a beginner's guide to help you start a clean eating habit. Be positive about it and form a support group. Learn from the people who have done it, and believe in yourself that you can do it, too. Listen to your body and do not starve yourself; understand that it is important not to quit along the way in order to reap the benefits. To sum it all up, do not stop exercising and eat clean meals. Clean eating can help with weight loss, but exercise is good for the body.

The Importance of Mindful Eating

There are different reasons that meal planning is significant. For starters, people utilize meal planning when they are focusing on various health and wellness goals. To survive, people need to eat. People are supposed to consume at least three meals in a day. As for health and fitness goals, some people want to lose weight. When formulating a meal plan, some of the major factors to consider include the presence of medical issues and allergies. The medical issues can be managed by ensuring that people have a healthy and good diet. Some of the major reasons that meal plans are important include the fact that they help people to save money. Also, meal planning ensures that people's food intake is controlled.

The person formulating the meal plan will get to know whether they are having a balanced diet. For instance, during each serving, there should be enough vegetables, fruits, and whole grains. To maintain a good weight, the best option is to have a controlled food intake. Meal planning also ensures that people can see that there is diversity in the types of food that they consume. The adults will also have major food requirements as compared to growing teens. Meal plans also ensure that people can keep track of what they consume daily or weekly.

Working With a Budget

Most people encounter some challenges when coming up with a food budget. Everyone has a different budget in mind, especially in a household that has numerous members. Some people will opt to spend a certain amount of money on foods that will align with their diet needs and goals. For instance, a vegetarian will formulate a budget that contains a lot of vegetables. After coming up with a meal plan, it is possible to buy things in bulk, and they usually save some significant amount of money in the process. The meal plan also ensures that you do not consume any type of food in an unplanned manner, and that way, you can lead a healthy life. For example, sometimes, people may find out that they do not have food in the house, and they will go ahead and buy some food from a restaurant. As for the meal plans, you will always have food in the house. You should also ensure that you have adhered to the meal plan without any setbacks.

When purchasing food in bulk, you may also get some discounts. The best storage method is ensuring that the food is kept in a frozen state. It is also possible to prepare a variety of meals when you have a meal plan. The highly varied menus come in handy, and you can also get to enjoy numerous delicacies throughout the week. For instance, you can replace oatmeal with various types of fruits. Your house will also be graced by a suitable scent. The dinner and lunch plans can also be adjusted accordingly. Although some people may prefer to consume different types of meals in a day, the meal plan will help them to eliminate the guess work that is present when they are trying to decide which type of food they should consume at a particular moment.

By now, you understand that a meal has to be palatable for it to be enjoyed. It also has to appeal to the appetite, and as such, elements such as colors, texture, taste, and the general appearance and presentation really matter. But the most important is that the meal is balanced. To have a properly balanced meal, there is a need to plan. Below, we outline some of the reasons that it is important to plan for your meals.

- Meal planning helps make the best use of resources, including time, budget, and even the food itself. For the food to meet the social, physical, and psychological needs of a family, it is important that the meals are properly planned. As such, the family members can stay strong, healthy, and free from nutritional deficiencies. There is also a proper economy on fuel, labor, and time when meals are planned as often; thorough consideration is put into what methods are being used to prepare the foods. Since they are tailored according to the family's budget, money can only be spent in the best ways, and a family can afford a balanced diet that suits their needs. Knowing exactly which foods the family will need and in what amounts is important.

- Also, as a person planning the meals, you will be equipped with knowledge regarding foods from the same food group, and, therefore, you will be able to select a different variety of meals without foods becoming monotonous. This variety is also important for nutritive value, as taking food from the same food group may deprive you of the other nutrients in the foods within a food group. This is, therefore, an important factor to consider when planning your meals. Children also like to watch parents as they plan and cook meals, and this can provide learning and bonding platform for both parties.

- Meal planning also helps families deal with the widespread issue of food wastage. Meal planning works against wastage because you will understand that the meal needs specific ingredients, and you will be clear on what needs to be purchased. When planning meals, you will find yourself purchasing only what you need, and you can use what is extra for another meal. For instance, if you were cooking supper, you could use some of what remains during lunch, or you could use ingredients that remained during preparation of another meal. For example, when making an omelet in the morning, it may be possible to make use of vegetables from the previous day.

- Meal planning can help in instilling discipline. This is because when you understand that you have to plan for meals, then you will reduce the tendency to make last-minute decisions about food. This new pattern of thinking can help you get in control of your eating habits, and over time, it can help reduce the stress you face when you have to make last-minute food decisions. As a bonus, this can result in adequate control of weight as you can control the portions you are served.

Chapter 10 Weight Loss – Nutrition, Calories, Macros and Micros

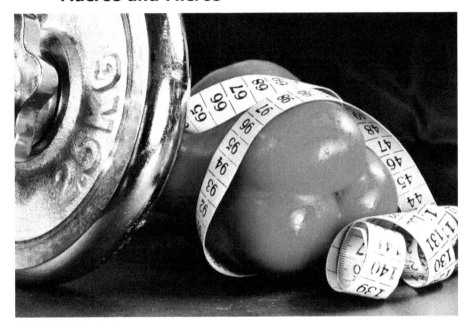

How weight loss works – with a personal story to match!

This will have to be a simplified version of the weight loss process! And keep in mind, not everyone is the same and some people lose weight more easily than others, and others may keep weight on for various health reasons. Make sure you see your doctor first if you are aiming to lose weight, as they can look through your medical history and point out any potential patterns or issues, which could help you to find the best method for you. Now that that's out of the way, we can get into the general rules and sciences behind weight loss.

So, when you eat food, you are taking in energy (calories). When you move and exercise, you are burning calories. When you burn more calories than what you are eating, you will lose weight. Keep in mind that your body needs a basic number of calories in order to survive and keep your organs running, which is why it's very important to eat enough. I add this because when I first started to consider calories I was a bit taken aback by the notion of "burning more calories than you take in", thinking I would have to burn 1800 calories worth of exercise a day! But perhaps that was just my very silly mistake; you are probably a lot more intelligent than that!

When you reach a calorie deficit, your body begins to turn to energy sources, which are already in your body, i.e. stored fat. Sometimes, muscle can also be used for energy, which does result in weight loss, but it also results in muscle loss and a less-toned physique. You can remedy this by incorporating strength training into your fitness routine, as well as high intensity cardio. By doing this, you are helping your body to burn fat as well as building muscle at the same time. You also need to eat properly to give your body enough protein and energy to get through those workouts and repair those muscles properly afterward!

Some people opt for the low-calorie method of weight loss, and I have also done that. It worked for a while but I couldn't sustain it, so I had to turn to another method. I decided to ramp-up my workouts and eat a more well-rounded diet, full of nutritious foods, and enough of them. By training with weights and high intensity cardio, my metabolism became faster and more efficient, and my increased muscle mass helped me to burn more calories.

Calories

"Calories" is basically another word for energy. When you eat, you are consuming energy, which your body uses to function and grow. If you eat too many calories, you will put on weight, if you reduce them, you will lose weight. You can figure out how many calories you need in order to lose weight by punching your weight, height, age, gender and activity level into an online calorie-counter. It will tell you how many calories you need to eat in order to lose, gain or maintain weight. A good rule of thumb is to reduce your calorific intake by 300-500. This can be done pretty easily just by cutting out high-calorie foods such as processed treats, cakes, ice cream, white starches and alcohol.

Macronutrients

Macronutrients are the main groups your food is categorized under: carbs, fats, and proteins. Each of these has a particular function in the body, and they are all important for weight loss and general health. I know there are many people out there who banish carbs, but let's make this book a carb-friendly zone!

Carbohydrates

Carbs give you energy! Your body adores carbs because it's an easy energy source. Carbohydrates, especially those found in starchy or sugary foods are often very high in calories, which is why people avoid overeating carbs when trying to manage their weight. When you don't burn off the energy you consume, your body stores it as fat – so it's best to eat a high-carb meal on days when you are active and exercising. As long as you eat carbs which come from whole, natural sources with slow-releasing energy, there's absolutely no need to fear them! If you want to eat bread? Opt for a wholegrain sourdough from a real bakery as opposed to a white loaf from the supermarket (these are often full of sugar and refined white flour). If you feel like pasta?

Opt for a whole-meal variety and take note of the serving size on the packet and stick to it so you don't add extra calories with large portions.

Carbs to eat:

- Starchy veggies such as sweet potatoes
- Fruits and berries
- Whole grains such as quinoa, brown rice, oats
- Wholegrain breads and pastas

Carbs to avoid:

- Processed, white flour (cakes and baked goods, white bread)
- White pasta
- White rice (in moderation is fine, but brown rice is far better)
- Sugary foods (sweets, cakes, ice cream...all of the classic sugary snacks!)

Fat

Healthy fats are important for the body to function properly. Fats make you feel satiated and full, and they help the body to absorb and process essential nutrients and proteins. Good fats found in foods such as fish and avocadoes are great for cognitive (brain) health and keeping the skin in good condition. Adding a source of healthy fat to your dinner will help you to feel satisfied. Opt for nuts, seeds, avocado, fish and olive oil.

Fatty foods to eat:

- Avocadoes
- Nuts and seeds
- Olive oil
- Oily fish such as salmon and tuna

Fatty foods to avoid:

- Fried foods (fast foods)
- Processed fats such as margarine

Protein

Protein is very important for muscle growth, that's why hard-core lifters are always guzzling protein shakes and egg whites! If we didn't eat any protein, our cells, bones, muscles, nails, (basically our whole body!) couldn't repair and renew itself and grow stronger. It's important to incorporate protein into your diet so your body can remain strong and supported. Protein is also very satiating so it fills you up and keeps cravings at bay.

Protein to eat:

- **Eggs**
- Lean red meat
- Lean chicken

- Fish
- Unsweetened yogurt
- Beans and lentils
- Tofu

Protein to avoid:

- **Fatty meats**

Micronutrients

Micronutrients are far more commonly known as vitamins and minerals. We usually take supplements and pills to boost our micronutrients, especially in the winter when we are prone to get sick. However, you really can get enough micronutrients through a proper diet (unless you have a condition which hinders your body's ability to absorb and hold onto certain micronutrients). As long as you eat lots of fresh fruits, veggies, lean meats, grains and seeds you should be getting enough micronutrients. However, blood tests can detect micronutrient deficiencies and you can take supplements to remedy this.

Important micronutrients to keep an eye out for:

- **Iron**
- Magnesium
- Folate
- Calcium

- Zinc
- B, A, C and E vitamins

Conclusion

After reading the entire book, the next step is to follow up on the meal plans that have been indicated in the context above. The meal planning guide will ensure that you have achieved all your needs. You may come up with a schedule that you will follow while also adhering to some of the guidelines that are present. Some tasks may seem somewhat complex; however, what matters most is the ability to breakdown each task into individual subtasks. The meal plan may seem silly to some; however, it will ensure that you can meet some of your goals, including leading a healthy lifestyle. After following up on the meal planning for beginners, at the end of it all, you will be glad that you followed up on the meal plan to the letter. Evidently, meal planning should provide a way to achieve various body goals regarding matters of health. At the same time, learners should be able to grasp a few basics related to the benefits of having a meal planning strategy. Other than that, it is going to be important for meal planning strategies to be incorporated into the lives of other consumers so that they are in a position to practice the routine and policies involved in the meal planning series.

With the chapters of this book, learners or beginners can successfully incorporate the basics of meal planning into their lives. They shall also be in a position to learn more about the health basics of leading a healthy life by incorporating a viable eating method. At the end of it all, it is going to take more than just reading these chapters to actually understand the benefits of learning more about the importance of meal planning. Being a beginner, you should now be in a position to actually grasp the most important details of meal planning in order to be in a position to help your children and other family members to incorporate the lessons into their schedules, too. Toward that end, by now, you should master the trends involved in the meal planning business.

After completing all the necessary preparations, it is essential to understand all the plans were part of a bigger plan, which may be leading a healthy lifestyle while also reducing weight progressively. To ensure that you have achieved your goals, you should ensure that you have adhered to the meal plans that have been provided in the above context. You must also be prepared to follow up on the provided meal plan. Now that you fully understand what it takes to be a successful meal planner, you can go ahead and take notes on your own practices when planning for your meals weekly and monthly.

With this book, you were able to learn more about what you have been missing in your daily life, which is to lose some weight. You were also able to grasp basic lessons on how vital it is to be a part of a world that is taking in new trends of eating and watching their weight. In the end, you will understand what it takes to become a responsible individual who watches the value of proper meal planning and portion control.

As you do your own meal planning, you shall understand what it takes to be in a position to make healthy meals every day of your life, as long as it contributes to your well-being. Apart from that, the text shared the basics of creating a reliable shopping list that you can go back to before you delve into a shopping spree for your list of ingredients. With the right list of groceries, you will learn to evade impulse buying, as well. You have also learned how to integrate meal planning, not only at home but also at the commercial sector. As you apply what you learned, you will embrace these lessons since they are vital elements of living a healthy, happy life.